FOREVER
One Pink LINE

A JOURNEY THROUGH FAILED IVF

SONJA ROOS

Forever, One Pink Line: A Journey Through Failed IVF
©Sonja Roos 2024

All rights reserved. No part of this book may be reproduced or used by any means, graphic, electronic, or mechanical, including photocopying, recording, taping, or by an information storage retrieval system without the expressed written permission of the copyright owner except in the case of brief quotations embodied in critical articles and reviews.

Copyright of the overall book production belongs to Aldwyn Rostant.

Because of the dynamic nature of the Internet, any web addresses or links contained here within may have changed since publication and may no longer be valid.

The stories and the lived experiences shared are those of the contributor alone. Some names and identifiable characteristics have been changed but do not diminish the history.

ISBN: 978-1-923163-42-3 (Paperback)
          978-1-923163-43-0 (eBook)

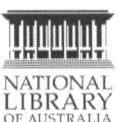 A catalogue record for this book is available from the National Library of Australia

Contents

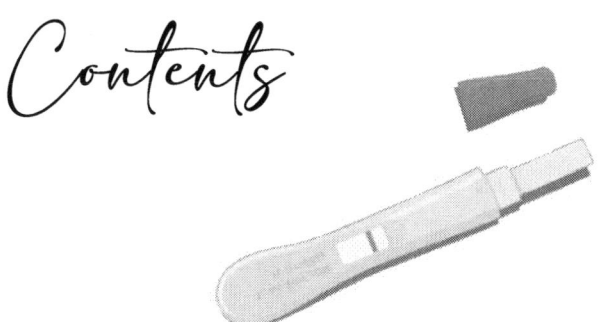

Preface v

Chapter 1	The beginning 1
Chapter 2	Trying to conceive 7
Chapter 3	The News 17
Chapter 4	The First Appointments 21
Chapter 5	The Process of IVF 27
Chapter 6	The Back-up Donor 29
Chapter 7	Round 1 35
Chapter 8	My 30th Birthday 45
Chapter 9	IVF – the 'gift' that did not stop giving 59
Chapter 10	Third time's the charm? 65
Chapter 11	Déjà vu 79
Chapter 12	When it all got too much 85

Chapter 13	The miracle	91
Chapter 14	Pregnant, not pregnant	97
Chapter 15	The last one	103
Chapter 16	Opting out	111
Chapter 17	Childless not by choice	117

Acknowledgements 121

Preface

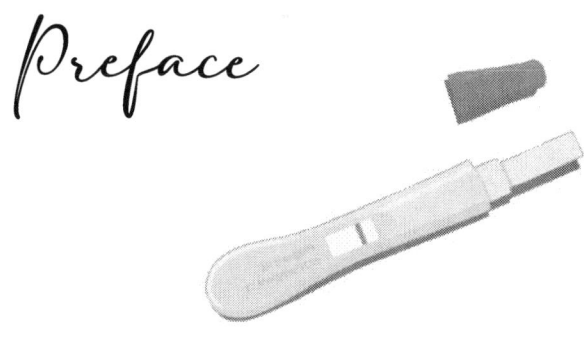

I AM AN AVID planner. My life is ruled by schedules, routines, and plans. I am not flexible, not even a little bit. I have also always felt the need to be in control. If I were in control, nothing could or would go wrong, right? Wrong! Infertility and our consequent childlessness was not part of my plan. You know that five- or ten-year plan you carefully set out in your mind? The plan that looks suspiciously like so many other people's plans? The plan that helps you fit in with society? Yeah, that plan.

My checklist (post high school) looked like this:

1. Study and get a good job.
2. Get married.
3. Have two kids at least three years apart and the first one no later than age thirty.
4. Become a part-time stay-at-home mum so I don't miss out on any milestones.
5. Eventually buy a house—the white-picket-fence kind with a big garden where the kids can play.
6. Live happily ever after.

The plan itself seemed simple and achievable on paper, but the reality of life is that everything does not always work out how you planned it, and you are stuck having to try to formulate a plan B.

This book is for every person stuck on having to formulate a plan B or even C. For every person who, despite going through multiple IVF treatments, still had to walk out empty-handed, be it due to finances, emotional limits, or any other reason. No-one gets to ask you why you gave up on treatments. Is giving up even the right word if you exhausted all the options you were comfortable with? I don't think so. You are one of the strongest people around. You held onto your dream and went through cycles of hope and devastation on repeat. You spent thousands of dollars and invested your entire being into your dream, but you have nothing to show for it. You are a warrior.

I want to tell everyone person going through infertility and involuntary childlessness that you are not alone. I know you feel alone and like no-one understands, and I still feel like that a lot of the time. Unfortunately, you can't make people understand how you feel; no-one can understand until they have stood in your shoes. There is no way to convey how it feels when you can't have the one thing you have always dreamed of. Even worse, there is no particular reason you can't have it. It isn't because you didn't try, are a bad person, or because you didn't work hard enough. Truth be told, you poured every ounce of your being into that dream, but the universe just decided that it was not in the cards.

This book is also for me. I want to raise awareness that IVF does not always equal a baby. I want to be honest with myself as to what I was feeling during the whole process and how I am feeling now after I have walked away from IVF: sad, broken, full of grief and, worst of all, empty-handed.

I am going to roll all the emotions out. No sugar-coating. No pulling up a veil pretending that I am okay with everything. No, it will be real, it will be messy, and it will be sad, but at the end, there will be a glimmer of hope on the way forward.

Here is our story.

Chapter 1

THE BEGINNING

I NEVER REALLY WANTED to wait long to have kids. I have always had this innate desire to be a mother. I absolutely adored children and spending time with them. My whole life I had this feeling that I was destined to be a mother, like it was the one and only purpose I had to fulfil in order to be "complete". It was also equally important for me to be financially stable before doing so.

I took a gap year after school and started pursuing a degree in law from the age of twenty. I enrolled in university in 2011. This was also the year I met my husband. He was a twenty-one-year-old civil engineering student and lived in the same apartment complex as me. I would never have thought that I would meet the love of my life there.

I am not going to bore you with our relationship stories. I will, however, bore you with how we met. In short, we bumped into each other outside our apartment building on the way to class and chatted for a few minutes. After our encounter, in typical girl fashion, I stalked him on social media, and a few weeks later, I plucked up the courage and sent him a cheesy message on Facebook. We have been together since.

One of the first questions my husband asked me was whether I had a child. Rude, I know. In his defence, I grew up in an area where pregnant high school girls weren't a big shock. I laughed at it back then. Now I just think it is really ironic, him wondering if I had a secret child while I was unknowingly infertile.

Like every young couple, we did not talk much about having children. I was also not keen on the idea of an accidental pregnancy back then. I drank my pill religiously every morning. It is a big joke now, thinking about how much money I spent on contraceptives. I am also a bit mad at how the pill gets pushed on young girls. I often wonder if I would have noticed my fertility issues earlier if it was not masked by the fake period that contraceptives bring.

Anyway, there was no way in hell we were going to become another university pregnancy statistic. No, we were responsible. During the university years, the topic of babies and kids was solely reserved for jokes. I loved to say to my husband, "I hope our kids get my self-discipline and your smarts," or "I think our kids will have my eyes because brown is a more dominant colour."

Now, just because I say we did not speak about it, that does not mean I did not dream about it in secret. Even during university, the dream of having children was there, whispering, as if from the other side of a door I was yet to unlock.

My husband finished his degree in 2014 and I finished mine in 2016. It was somewhere during this period that the desire for marriage and children started to become pretty strong, but the timing was not right. Frustratingly, there was no set plan for marriage yet. However, there was talk of immigrating to Australia. Although this scared me, I knew it would be better for our future children.

In January 2017, I started my first job, and in April 2017, we made the decision to start the immigration process. I was excited at the prospect that I could give our kids a better future there. We wanted to raise them in an environment where they were safe, could thrive, and would have ample opportunities—something that South Africa could not offer.

By February 2018, we got married and jetted off to Thailand for our honeymoon. I remember people telling me to "not go and get pregnant" on our honeymoon. The joke was on them, although nobody knew. I must admit I would not exactly have been disappointed if I did have a "whoops" on our honeymoon. Knowing my husband did not share this idea, I stuck with my religious pill-drinking ritual and had fun "practising" to make babies. Damn, if practice was all it took.

As soon as we arrived back from our honeymoon, I wanted to start trying for a family. There was no reason not to. Wrong! My husband seemed to be able to crush my dreams with little snippets of reality and practicality, which is probably a good thing but not always appreciated. The brakes were turned on with "no, not yet" or he was not ready yet or "it is not a good time". I loved to kick back with responses like "you will never be ready" and "there is never a good time". I lost the battle and we decided to wait after we immigrated. It was no big deal. I was only twenty-seven; I still had plenty of time to have kids, right?

Our permanent residency visas were granted in October 2018, and in December 2018, we packed up our old life and travelled a long way towards a future that would be better for our hypothetical children.

Getting edgy, it did not take me long to raise the question again. Needless to say, I lost the battle again in the face of practicality and logic. I let it go. I told myself that it was going to be the last time that I let it be. My husband might not have a biological clock, but mine was counting down the ticks. I was twenty-eight, and I knew that egg quality plummets from age thirty, at least if you are a person of average anatomy.

In February 2019, my mum passed away. Losing her felt like losing a small part of myself. I was especially upset at the idea that our children would never be able to meet her. Just the other day, I found a book she left me with the words *To my grandchild, love Grandma R.* I want to tear up just writing it down. I still keep that book tucked away, but I rarely take it out. It just reminds me of the two things I have lost.

Aside from my mum's passing, 2019 treated us well. We settled into our new country and jobs, made friends, and grew as people. Life was good, and to my surprise, my husband agreed that we could start trying to conceive in 2020.

I was the epitome of excitement. We were going to have a child.

Every time I thought about it, I grinned from ear to ear. Now, if you need to know anything about me, it is that I like to know things so I can plan and set expectations. This was no different. Google became my new best friend as I embarked upon a plethora of research.

First topic on the list: "Hey, Google, how long does it take for your period to return after stopping the pill?" This was a question that had been burning at the back of my mind for quite some time. I harboured some concern as I had been on the pill since the age of sixteen, so a good twelve years by the time I asked the question. Google did not disappoint with the answer. Then again, Google always backs you up, regardless of your argument. There will always be at least one more person who shares your position, and you only need that one. I felt relief when I read the first result. Research showed that it didn't matter how long you were on the pill, your normal period should come back within three months, and who was I to argue with Google?

Satisfied with this answer, I proceeded with the next question. "How long does it take to fall pregnant after stopping the pill?" Yet again, Google supported my naive thinking, stating it takes about three months, but some women are lucky enough to fall pregnant within the first month. I was filling up on hope and fast; I just did not realise it was false hope. Then again, my sister got pregnant in about three to four months after she stopped her pill. These things run in the family, right, so I should be pregnant by mid-2020.

Armed with this new knowledge, I confided in a few friends about our plans to start a family. I remember sitting at a kitchen table and excitedly telling them about our plans. Stories were exchanged of woman who got pregnant quickly after stopping the pill, and I was filled to brim with hope and reassurance that I had nothing to worry about.

A fond memory of that time was one of our friends saying that he could almost see me standing with a wooden spoon in the driveway and my husband running away with one kid on the hip and the other by the hand. I still smile when I think about it. The smile is different now. I used to smile at the prospect of the reality of it. Now, it is more a smile of sadness, of a life I will not have.

The year ended almost as quickly as it had started and, before I knew it, 2020, and the time to start trying to conceive, was upon us.

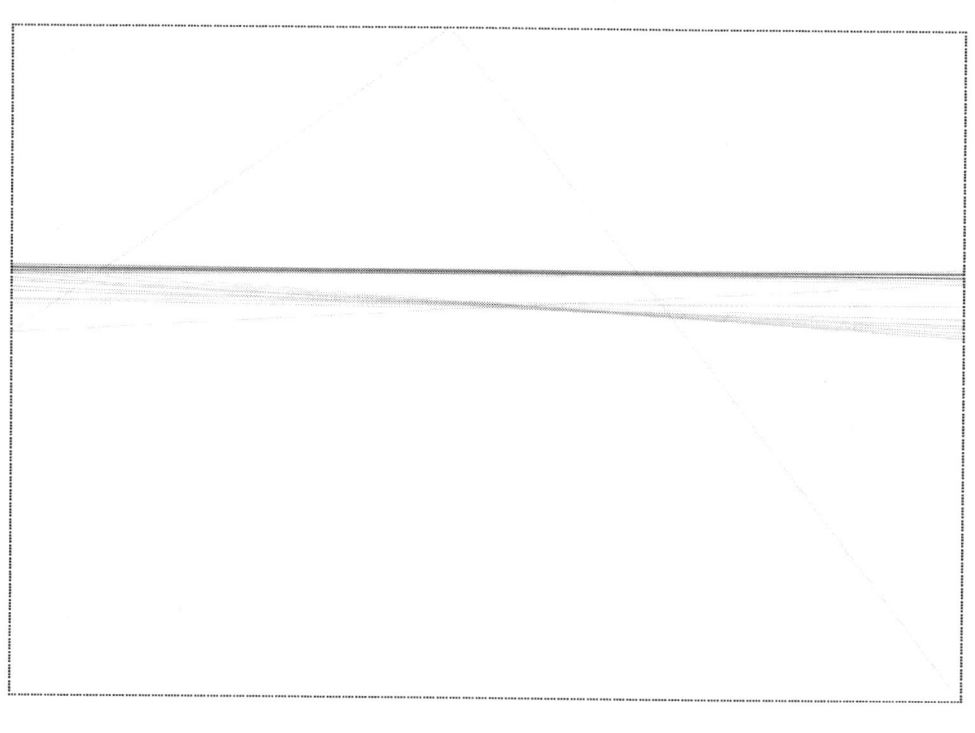

Chapter 2

TRYING TO CONCEIVE

WE DID NOT START trying immediately, although the desire was there. We had planned a trip home to South Africa for that February, and there was no use trying to get pregnant before we jetted off. *What if I got pregnant?* I thought. I didn't want to be on a flight while pregnant. I can almost hear the fertility gods saying, "Yeah, right," to the absurd idea of me getting pregnant within a span of two months.

In early February 2020, we set off to South Africa to see our friends and family after a very exciting year living in a new country. I could not wait to see my best friends and my family. I had this itch to tell them about our plans of starting a family. Unsurprisingly, they were just as excited about it as me. It was almost a "girly squeal" moment. Even more excited was my sister; she was happy that she was going to be an aunt and that her kids would finally have nieces and nephews. We talked about possible baby names and whether I would be a stay-at-home mum or working mum. You know, the usual things. Thinking back, it all seemed relatively simple. Sex Education 101: have sex, get pregnant, get baby. Looking at my luck and track record in life, I should have known that things would be everything but simple, but I didn't. No, I was living in a world made up of rainbows, unicorns, glitter, and butterflies. The perfect, very unrealistic world most of us wished was real.

After two and a half weeks, we headed home. I left in my glitter-filled bubble with a promise to friends and, of course, the sister that I would call them once I was pregnant. They are still waiting for that call. They did, however, get another kind of call a few months later, but we will get to that a little bit later.

Around the end of March, I finished the last of my contraceptive pills. The morning I popped the last one in my mouth, I felt elated, like anything was possible. Unfortunately, this "anything is possible" was going to come and bite me in the behind in the next few months.

We officially started trying in April 2020. Deep down, I knew it was too soon—I was barely off the pill. We were even so bold as to decide on some names for our children. Peyton for a girl and Daxton for a boy. My husband even created Gmail addresses for future them. It was like reserving a spot for them in our future.

Obviously, we did not anticipate anything going wrong with our clearly set and bookmarked plan. Why would we? It was drilled into us from an early age that if you had sex just once you will get pregnant. We were taught to use a condom and the pill because you can still get pregnant if you are just on the pill. In our current situation, I am just thinking, *Yeah, right, and flying pigs are real.* The idea of being able to get pregnant by having sex just once is comical to say the least.

The first month passed. Ambitiously, I took a pregnancy test. Of course, it was negative. What did I expect? My cycle was not even back to normal yet. I don't even think I told my husband about taking a pregnancy test. No need for both of us to be disappointed.

Even with no pregnancy on the horizon, I planned how I was going to tell him I was pregnant. It wanted it to be special and unique but not cheesy. Sometimes I would catch myself daydreaming of what colour the nursery would be and what it would look like.

The second month rolled around. You guessed it: another test, another negative. Once again, I tossed it in the bin and got on with life. It had only been two months.

We upped the number of times we were trying a week but not so much that it dictated our lives. I didn't want to schedule sex because that was certainly one way of taking the fun out of it.

I was also getting worried as my period was still AWOL. Can you get pregnant if you don't have a period? I knew that the answer was a hard no. I however was very happy taking up residence on planet denial. I did not want to let the thought that something might be wrong enter my mind for even a millisecond.

The months went by. Every month a pregnancy test. Every month a negative. I started to become discouraged, dreading to pee on that stupid, judgemental stick. I started feeling like a failure. Like I was a failure because I didn't conceive in the allotted time frame prescribed by Google. I am not sure how many tests I took before I let my husband enter my little world of insecurity and doubt. I voiced the little thoughts that had been lurking in the deep concerns of my mind:

"What if we can't have kids?" I knew I had the habit of getting anxious over small things and over-obsessing. Maybe this was one of those times. Regardless, my husband reassured me that everything was fine and that I should not worry. He sounded convincing, but I needed cold, hard facts. To do this, I visited a general practitioner to put my theory, that something was absolutely wrong, to the test.

I sat nervously in the waiting room. I could hear the clock ticking away in the background. Was it ticking down the time until I would get the most dreadful news ever? No, not yet. Sitting there, my mind was being overwhelmed by ideas including not being able to have children and, worse, being the reason that my husband would not be a dad. These thoughts very quickly escalated to whether he would leave me or what if something was seriously wrong, like some sort of disease? Like I said, I love overthinking; it is one of my least favourite pastimes, yet I engage in it at every possible opportunity. Sitting there with all those thoughts, I was on the verge of tears. It was as if all my thoughts were on a train, running on a rickety, never-ending track, the train heading towards a concrete wall with the inevitable outcome of crashing and burning.

Finally, the doctor called me into her rooms. I poured my heart out, but also stayed with the facts. I told her how we had been trying for more than three months and, more concerning, my period had not returned. I gave her the normal rundown of my family history and I was yet again filled with hope and reassurance that it will happen. She ordered a few tests just to be safe but regarded them as "really not that necessary". I was sent for an ultrasound and blood tests. We tested every possible relevant hormone level, down to iron levels. The one thing we did not test, however, was the most important one: my ovarian reserve, but we will get to that.

What were the results, you may ask. They were just peachy. Everything was 100% normal and I was probably just "stressed". Like I have not heard that before. Ugh, society forever blaming stress when they can't find a real reason for something. Yeah, yeah, I get it, I stress a lot about silly and insignificant things. I can't rewire my brain to not stress. The eggs and sperm will just need to get their shit in order and work around the stress. At that moment, another intrusive thought entered: *What if I won't be a good mum if I stress too much?* So, now I was stressing about stressing—great!

At twenty-eight years old, I sat by the phone like a fifteen-year-old girl waiting for a boy to call. At least, that is what it felt like. When the phone rang, I hesitated to answer. This was the moment, I thought. I wanted to know whether I was broken or not, whether I was a failure, but yet I also did not want to know. Talk about internal struggles. Knowing they would just call again, I took a deep breath and answered. I could feel a sense of relief washing over me, the tension in my shoulders dropping. The words "everything looks normal and within normal range" were the most beautiful words that I have ever heard. There was nothing physically wrong with me; I was normal. My husband gave me that "I told you so" look, and we plodded along.

Even though I knew there was nothing wrong with me, it still felt like something was off. It is hard to explain, like in a bad horror movie where a person has the feeling that someone is watching them, following them, but every time they turn around, they are alone. Yet the feeling of someone being there never goes away until the villain comes out to play. To me, infertility was the villain, and it was biding its time.

During the months we were actively trying, I called my sister—the same sister that was waiting for the "Hey, I'm pregnant!" call. Surprise—I was not. Like many others, she told me to just be patient. Ugh, I hated hearing those words. If she only knew I was on the verge of throwing something at her, she might have chosen different words. Yet she didn't know. I could not blame her for what she did not know. Not that I did not try. I might not have said my thoughts out loud, but I was solidly thinking, *What the hell does she know? It only took her a few months to conceive.*

I am not sure when it happened. Somewhere between all the crazy, something very annoying started to happen. Everywhere I went, I saw babies. Work, shopping centres, the park, commercials—you name it. It just did not stop. I just wanted to yell, "STOP!" as loudly as I could. It felt like the whole world was mocking me and my inability to conceive. My blood started to boil every time people complained about their kids and how hard it was to be parents. How dare they complain! Did they not realise what miracles kids are? Ungrateful much?!

Now, I have never known anyone who could not have kids, or perhaps I did and I was just oblivious to the fact. I knew I needed to know even if I did not want to. Against my better judgement, I typed the word *infertility* into my search engine. The page finished loading with multiple results. Summing up all of them, I got the following definition: *infertility means not being able to get pregnant after one year of trying (or six months if the woman is 35 or older).*

Screw Google, assuming from the outset that I am the problem, despite not being thirty-five yet. Tossing my phone on the bed, I walked to the mirror, sticking my stomach out to get an idea of how I would look when I was pregnant. I really wished it was real. I could feel the tears welling up in my eyes, but I blinked them away. This was stupid. Yet the idea of being infertile was eating me up from the inside. What if I couldn't be a mum? The thought sunk in, but I did not process it. I did the adult thing and buried it like a champion. If you can't see it, it does not exist, right? There was no way I was infertile. Infertility does not happen to people like us. Infertility happens to other people. How we as humans like to convince ourselves that nothing bad will happen to us because we are good people.

Around our fourth month of trying to conceive, a couple of our friends announced that they were pregnant. *Whoop-dee-doo*, I thought to myself, *congratu-fucking-lations for having sex and it actually working.* I obviously did not say this. What type of friend would I be? I swallowed my anger, sadness, and jealously and wrote a text with something along the line of *Congratulations, I am so happy for you guys.* I died a little bit on the inside that day. Little did I know how many times I would send that message in the next three years and how much more it would hurt every time.

It was early August 2020 and there was no period and no pregnancy. I once had this delusional thought that the pregnancy tests were all faulty. Ha, imagine that. Not getting or being pregnant despite trying for over five months and then telling yourself it is the pregnancy test's fault. If I was a little more delusional, I might have actually believed myself.

This was when self-blame started to set in. I started blaming my diet, my exercise, my stress, long work hours. I found every possible reason I could to explain why we didn't get pregnant. In reality, the reason was none of the above.

I had feelings of sadness, disappointment, and depression. I do not know if my husband harboured the same feelings. I would have preferred if he shared these feelings. I might have felt a little bit less alone if he had.

We were not quite at the one-year mark to be classified as "infertile", but around the middle of August 2020, my husband decided to have himself checked out. It couldn't hurt. We were pretty sure nothing was wrong. I mean, how often do you hear that men are the problem when it comes to fertility? Even the internet says, *When the **woman** is over/under 35*. We proceeded with the plan and off he went for a sperm analysis.

He was quite nervous about his results. He confided in me, saying that he thought he might have an issue. I am not going to go into detail, but there was a genuine concern. I shook it off and told him it would be fine, not unlike he did when I was worried about my issues. I told him that I loved him no matter what, and we left it at that. The test results were due in a week, so we waited.

I can't remember the specific date, but I can remember that it was a Thursday, it was an office day. He was particularly quiet that day. I did not make much of it, as sometimes he had a lot of meetings. I went about my day and came home at 5 pm.

I arrived home, turning the key in the lock, not knowing my life was about to do a 360. As I entered the house, he gave me a hug. It was a different hug than usual. Something was off, I could feel it. He was crying. Could that be? I have only ever seen him cry once before in the nine years we have been together.

"What's wrong?" I asked him. I expected him to tell me that a family member or a close friend had died. Maybe he lost his job. Did the doctor say he has some sort of terminal disease? All of the possible reasons ran through my mind. The actual reason was, once again, none of the above.

He opened his mouth, tears in his eyes, and said the words that would change both of our lives forever: "Would you still want to be with me if I shoot blanks?"

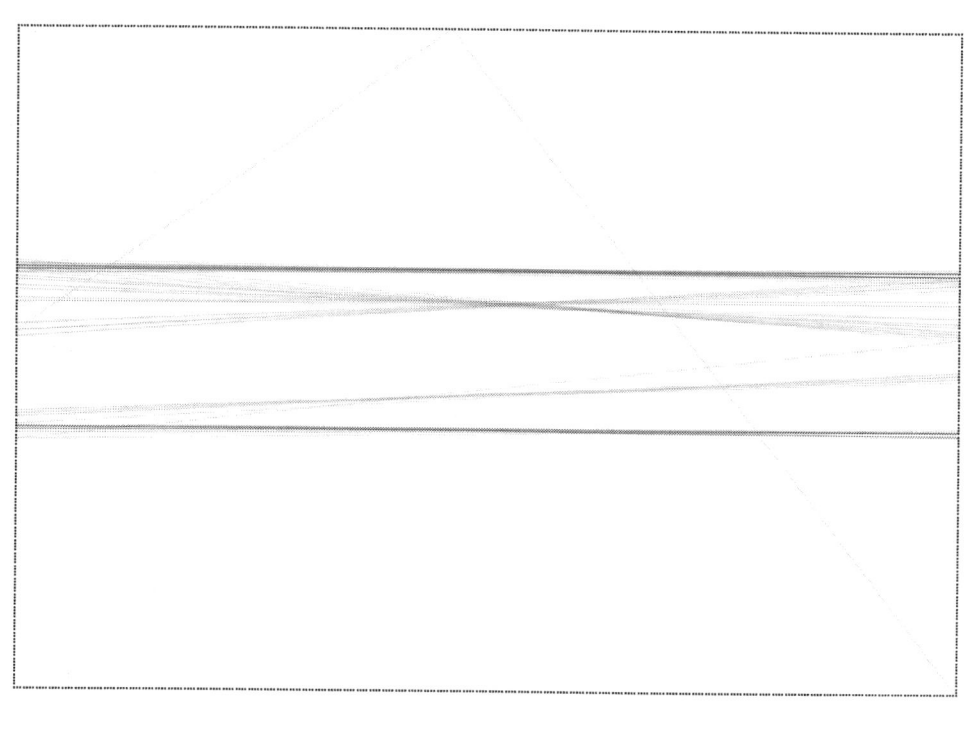

Chapter 3

THE NEWS

STUNNED AND DUMBFOUNDED, I did not know what to say. Did I hear him right? No, it could not be, could it? I gave him a hug and told him I loved him no matter. Honestly, saying those words, even though I meant every single one of them, killed me on the inside. I was still not 100% sure where he was getting this information from. We didn't know anything yet; his results were not even back yet. Was this his nervousness surfacing? Certainly not.

We sat on the couch and, a little more calmly, he told me that his results were actually back. His sperm analysis came back. The result: a big, fat ZERO.

Zero sperm. That is ridiculous. He was a man; men had sperm. How could he not have any sperm? I was having trouble processing this new information.

As we sat on the couch, a thought sprang to mind: IVF. Lots of people have children through IVF. It's easy. IVF equals baby. Problem solved. My husband agreed that there might be some options. At that stage, I had clearly forgotten that you still need sperm to make a baby and he had no sperm. However, I don't recall either of us making mention of it.

We decided to make an appointment with our general practitioner as a first step. While we waited for the first appointment, I took the time going in circles as to why the results were impossible. I searched the internet and annoyingly only got links to medical terms I did not understand. I was lost, upset, scared, and uncertain. I also wanted to be supportive towards my husband. I mean, he was the one who got the news. Unfortunately, I did not really know how to support him. I did not know what he needed. He probably just needed some space. I, on the other hand, needed solutions. There was no way that I would not be able to have a child, and the doctor would surely offer me viable solutions.

Our doctor confirmed that my husband's sperm count was a big, fat zero. He said my husband had a condition called azoospermia. He continued to say that the condition had two versions. A fixable, obstructive version and then the non-obstructive kind which you can't fix by way of medical intervention. He stated that we would likely need to go the IVF route if my husband had non-obstructive azoospermia. I could feel tears stinging my eyes, some of them rolling down my cheeks. My husband was sent for an ultrasound; the result would set our fate regarding IVF in stone.

The ultrasound was done that afternoon, and the devastating news on non-obstructive azoospermia hit us right in the balls, so to speak. The reality of having to do IVF hit soon thereafter. I wanted to scream from the rooftops how unfair all of this was. I was spiralling, thoughts whirling around me as if I was stuck on the inside of a tornado, dark thoughts pressing in from the outside, squeezing me. Thoughts like *What did we do to deserve this? We are good people; why do people who do drugs get to have kids and we can't? I am never going to experience how to conceive a baby naturally, I will never know the excitement of trying to conceive and then seeing those two pink lines on a stick.* It is safe to say that I was having a full-blown pity party. Balloons, cake, and all.

After I had calmed down as much I possibly could in such a situation, I started wondering how we were going to get through it. The idea of IVF terrified me. I am no good with needles. I basically go into a freak-out, panic mode every time I need to get blood drawn. How was I going to inject myself? I knew I would do it for my husband, I just didn't know how.

I called my dad but really wanted my mum at that moment. I don't know if my dad was holding back emotion or whether he was just being his usual practical self, but he basically told me that he was sorry, but it was good that we had the IVF backup plan. Hanging up the phone, I could not stop thinking about how useless the conversation was. I didn't feel better. Maybe I should have called my sister instead. She is a woman; she would understand. Wrong again. How could she possibly understand? Listening, she asked me if I was okay. How I dislike those words. My husband likes to say that if you are not bleeding, you are okay. I have never quite agreed with that reasoning. There are so many things in life that would make you be "not okay". At that very moment, I was everything but okay. I was sad and terrified. I did not tell my sister this. I did the adult thing—swallowed my feelings and told her that I was okay and I would give her an update soon. By this time, I had had two useless conversations for the day. I kept to myself for the rest of my night, throwing yet another pity party. I should have been more grateful that we could afford IVF, but I was more focused on the unfairness of it all.

The next day, I took it upon myself to find a fertility specialist. How do you choose a person? Looking at the options, it was like saying, "Which of these people look like they will be able to give me a child?" All of them were probably qualified enough, but we, or rather I, picked Dr B. We were scheduled to see doctor in two weeks' time.

How many breakdowns can I person have in two weeks, you may wonder. The answer is at least five. I even had one at work. All sense of professionalism and keeping it together went out the door. The breakdowns were inevitable, though. I was so stressed, nervous, anxious, scared, uncertain, and angry that it all just bubbled over. I confided in a colleague who suggested I go home. I decided to work through it. I was an adult, for heaven's sake. I was not going to be put in a timeout just because I had a moment of weakness. Looking back, I should probably just have taken the day.

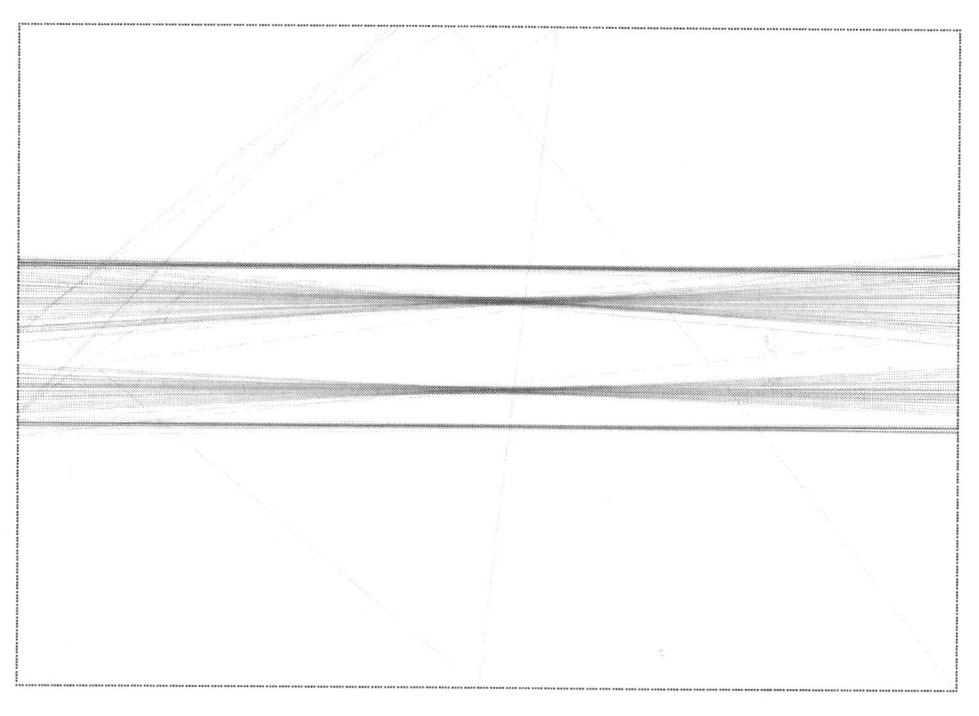

Chapter 4

THE FIRST APPOINTMENTS

ON 9 SEPTEMBER 2020, we had our first fertility appointment. Who would have thought three years earlier that we would end up here? Definitely not me. I went my whole life, twenty-nine years of it, to be exact, believing that I could achieve anything if I just put enough hours in and worked hard. Nothing I have ever done has proven to be contrary to this theory. That is until infertility happened.

Up until that moment, my personality of planning, determinism, self-discipline, and perfection had helped me achieve many things in my life. I excelled in athletics in primary school and became prefect of the year. In high school, I got top notch grades and prided myself in being in the academic top ten. Yet I couldn't make a baby by putting in the time and effort.

Sitting in the fertility clinic, waiting for our first appointment, I felt like I was going to throw up from nervousness. My husband held my hand as he was preoccupied with his own thoughts. Dr B called us into his rooms. He seemed so positive as he sat us down.

We talked a little bit about the situation. You know, the one where we were reproductively screwed and needed to use other means. As my tests were normal, we focused on my husbands' fertility challenges. Dr B had a whole lot of things to say that day, but they all kind of blurred into one another. From what I could understand at the time, my husband had non-obstructive azoospermia and that we could still get sperm from him using an operation called a microTESE. This procedure was successful in retrieving sperm, "but", he added—oh, why did there always have to be a *but?*—there were no guarantees.

No guarantees. Here I thought IVF would magically give me a baby and this guy can't even give me a 100% foolproof way to extract sperm from my husband. To add to the already unconventional circumstances, the doctor decided to sprinkle a little extra surprise on top of it all. We were not prepared for the words "back-up donor". *Say what, now?!* is the response I wanted to give, but instead, I gave him something that I presume was a blank stare. Leaving us to mull that over, the doctor turned his attention to me.

At first, he sounded pretty confident that we had nothing to worry about from my perspective. Then the dreaded period question came, and concern set in as soon as I told him I had been off the pill for six months with no period. Going into panic mode, I asked whether this could be due to being on the pill for ten years. Disappointingly, he said no. My heart sank, but I didn't say much. I felt like I shouldn't. What my husband was going through was much worse than not getting your period. Gosh, many women would be grateful for not having a period.

Despite the doctor telling us that we couldn't fix my husband and that we might need to consider donor sperm and that there might be more issues due to me not getting a period, he seemed surprisingly positive. He was certain that we would be able to get pregnant through IVF.

We were sent for more tests and went on our "merry" way.

Getting into the car, I hated the entire world. This was too much to process. I just wanted to scream that this was not okay; it was not okay that we had to pay to get what other people got to get for free. My husbands' words—"It is what it is"—infuriated me. How could he be so calm? "It is what it is". Really? Was that how he really felt? Burying my anger, I tried to find a way to bring up the small detail of a back-up donor. As much as I wanted to avoid it, we couldn't.

My husband, on the other hand, had a very different approach in mind. He proceeded to take the topic, put it in a little boxed room in his mind and bolted the iron-clad door shut with a million locks. There was no way we were going to discuss this if he could help it. Any discussion was going to lead to an argument, and oh boy, did we have arguments.

I've read in the past that infertility can make or break your marriage. It can either make you stronger as a couple, or the stress and trauma of it all can break you apart. Taking the above circumstances into account, I can vouch for both. My husband and I are stronger, but there were also times when I was not sure whether our relationship would survive. Discussing the possible donor was one of these times. The conversation about whether he wanted a child enough that he would let go of his genetics was a sensitive one. I knew it was more important to him than it ever was to me. This scared me. Did he love me enough and did he want a child enough that he could let go of the desire for a biological child? I was afraid to know the answer. The donor argument was put on hold for the time being, but I knew the "peace" would not last forever.

Our follow-up appointment came. I was not sure why I dreaded it; how much worse could our situation really get? It already felt like we got the raw end of the bargain, like the fertility gods fucked us over. Like the universe had it in for us. There is nothing that the doctor could say that could make me feel worse. Surprise! I was wrong again. At this point, I should probably have stopped going with my gut feeling; it clearly had no instinct.

So, guess what? There was indeed something that could make things worse. Adding insult to injury, Dr B uttered the words "low AMH for your age". I did not know what he meant, but it certainly did not sound like something to celebrate. Bringing it down to basics, it meant that my ovarian reserve was low for someone who was only twenty-nine years old. In other words, if you want a baby, you should probably get on it soon—you have less time than you thought.

I just sat there. I remember my husband reaching for my hand and, as if there was a trigger button on my hand, soft tears spilled from my eyes. You could almost see the pity in the doctor's eyes and the sadness in my husband's as a tissue was handed to me. As per usual protocol, I was reassured that although my AMH was low, we still had a chance, it was just a little bit lower. Staying positive, I see.

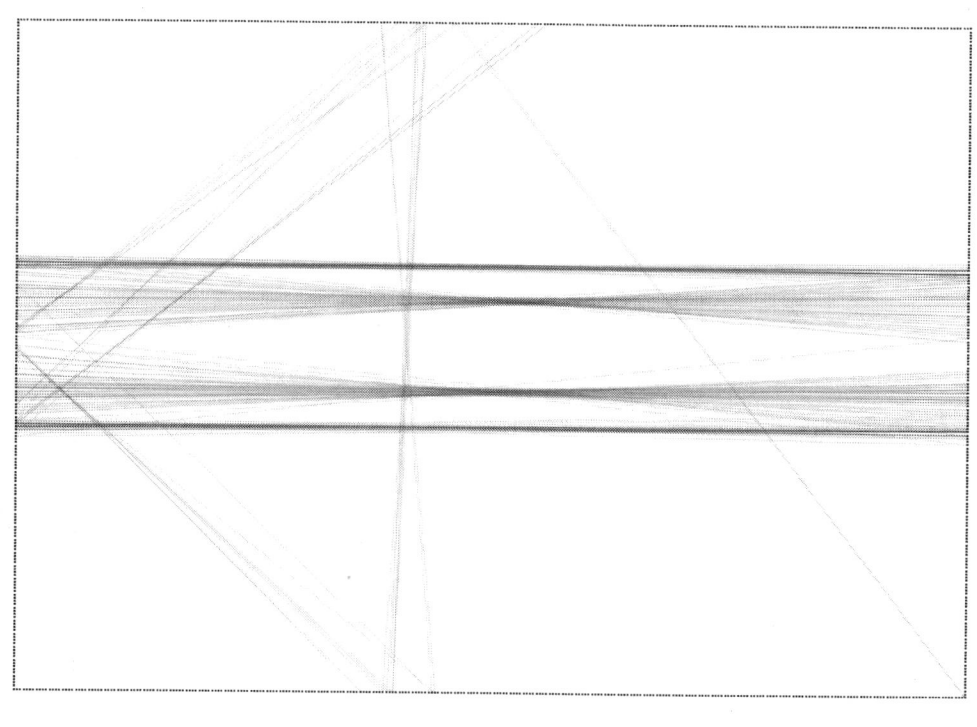

Chapter 5

THE PROCESS OF IVF

DURING THE CONSULTATION, THE "relatively simple" process of IVF was explained. Summed up, I would need to inject myself with at least two needles a day for fourteen days. In those fourteen days, I would have to do multiple check-ups and blood tests and be prodded with an internal vaginal ultrasound. Then we would do an egg-collection procedure. These eggs, if mature, would be fertilised with sperm (either my husband's or a donor's) to make embryos, and then they would put an embryo back in me on day three or five and hope it sticks. Like I said, "relatively simple". Almost like having sex—totally the same thing.

I could not stop thinking about how horrible it all sounded. It felt like I was on a game show and the host was announcing that we had just won the infertility lottery. No sperm, no period, low AMH. The prize? We get to spend a fortune on trying to have a baby and inject ourselves with needles—yay!

I wanted to punch something or someone—it did not really matter who or what. I was angry at the fact that we got dealt a shitty hand and I was sad. To put it in the words of Oh, a character from the movie *Home*, I was sad-mad.

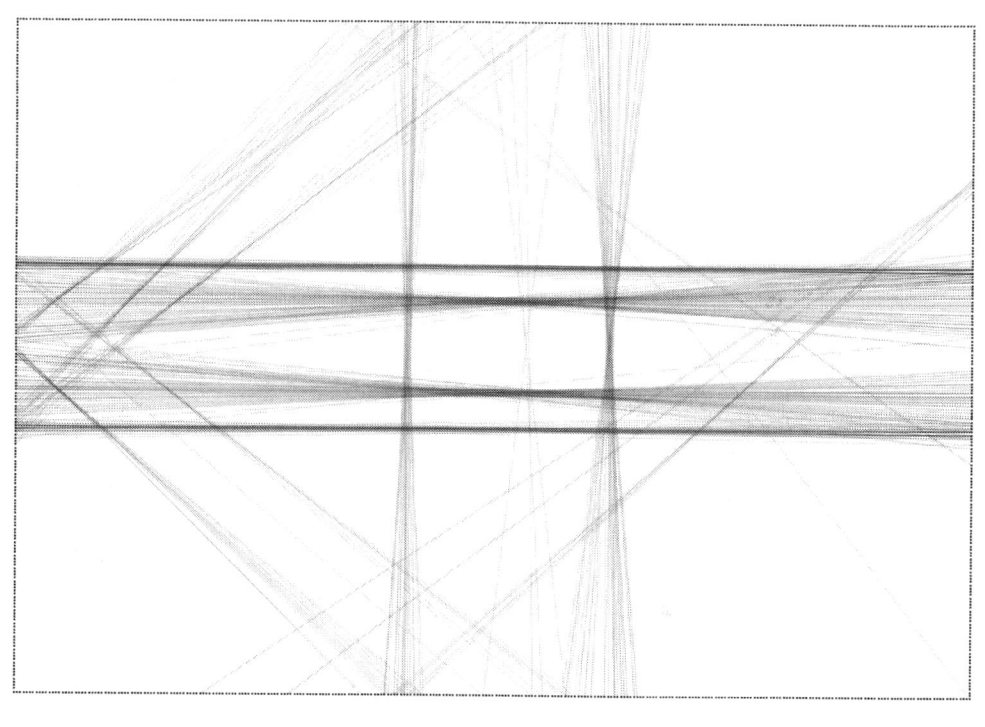

Chapter 6

THE BACK-UP DONOR

AS WE APPROACHED OUR first IVF round, we had to start thinking about a back-up donor. At one stage, my husband wanted to use his father's sperm. You could just imagine my reaction. Hell no! The idea was weird, and I just couldn't. I just could not imagine having my father in law's ingredients in me. The idea freaked me out. It was too weird. Don't get me wrong. I love my father-in-law. He is an amazing man, but there was no way I was having his biological child. What if it worked? Would he then be grandpa-dad? I know my husband was just trying to cling onto his genetic material for dear life.

To my relief, we did not go with this option. The major factor was probably just me giving a hard, no-argument no. The other argument was that his dad was older and had already had a vasectomy. An anonymous donor was the route to go.

With much convincing needed, my husband agreed for us to look at back-up donor sperm. The first step was to get counselling. I did not understand what the big deal was at that stage. It was only sperm, right? As time went by, I did start to contemplate the direct and indirect implications of using a donor, but more about that later.

We underwent the counselling, consisting very much of us telling our story and the counsellor asking us questions. The counsellor also explained to us the difference between using a known donor vs an anonymous one and the legal and other implications. It was a lot of information to take in, but I was all-in. If my husband did not have sperm, we needed a back-up, and I was okay with that.

Looking back, I was being really insensitive towards my husband's feelings and what he needed. I was selfish because I really wanted a family with him, and I did not try to put myself in his shoes to understand what he was feeling.

He looked fine with everything, and every time I tried to ask him about it, he closed up, or worse, he would say, "It is what it is." It was difficult to understand that he was having a hard time with it when he didn't open up to me about it. I don't think it would have changed much even if I did know. I was so focused on "having a solution" that I simply did not care about anything else. I was going to have my family at all costs. Selfish, I know.

After the counselling, we got sent a link to donors. It was an odd feeling scrolling through the list. It felt like "shopping" for my child's biological father. It is a cruel way to put it, as no child should feel like they were just bought as part as some sort of transaction. I don't know how to explain it in a different way, though. You had a list of numbers, with a baby picture and a profile of each. The profile contained physical characteristics, hobbies, careers, interest, medical history, and some familial history.

None of these people however seemed to fit the bill. How do you choose someone to replace your partner, so to speak? None of these people were him. I was looking for a replica—a doppelganger, if you will. Deep down, I knew I would not find such a thing. We had to settle for less. Someone who might not look like my husband but who had similar characteristics. Just before I came to the end of the donor list, feeling quite defeated, I came across a donor; he was a similar height to my husband with the same hair colour. He was analytical and liked hanging out with friends. His profile said he was responsible, value-driven, and self-disciplined. Furthermore, just like my husband, he stated that he could get tied up in details and not see the bigger picture. Even better, he was an Afrikaner, South African. It felt like a sign.

I felt like he was the donor for us. My heart immediately stopped when I saw he only had the capacity to make one more family. For completeness, I should mention that each donor is only able to make ten families.

My husband was still working while I screened donors. I, on the other hand, had forgotten that I actually have a real job. I had given myself the new job of finding our donor. My real job was not extremely high on my priority list, but I did not let it suffer, either. We were both working from home that day and I tried getting him to come and look at the profile.

Unsurprisingly, he was refusing. He felt like I was pushing him into a corner to decide. I was probably doing it, but not on purpose. I was very well-intentioned. I knew that we would not be able to get a donor better than that, and my argument was that we probably wouldn't use it anyway—it was just a back-up.

After some arguments and tears, my husband agreed to look at it, but we were not reserving it just yet. He wanted to talk to his parents about the potential donor. What the fuck did they have to do with it? It is not their choice! I was seething but let it go, sort of. He arranged an impromptu video call with his parents in South Africa to work through the options we had sharing our computer screen with them, and although being supportive, it did not sound like they were 100% on board with the idea. You know, how could I expect my husband to raise another man's child?

This made me so livid. It was not another man's child. My husband would be the dad. What makes a dad is being there for a child and raising them, not giving sperm. Anyone could be a father, but it takes a special person to be a dad. How could none of them see it?

After some deliberation and my husbands' parents likely realising the gravity of the situation—that this might be the only opportunity for them to ever become grandparents—they agreed that from the available options, the donor we chose was by far the best of the lot.

This was one of the most difficult moments I've ever seen my husband go through, even if I didn't grasp the extreme importance of the decision and what it meant to him and his family. I could hear in my father-in-law's voice that he was struggling with the situation as well. I can't remember the exact words he used, but it was along the lines of "We should be grateful that we have the opportunity and modern medicine that can help make this dream of ours come true."

We went on and reserved two vials of sperm. By the way, sperm is ridiculously expensive. It was like another punch to the gut. Once again, we had to pay for something that other people got for free.

With the donor sperm on ice, we were ready for the first round of IVF, or at least as ready as we would ever be.

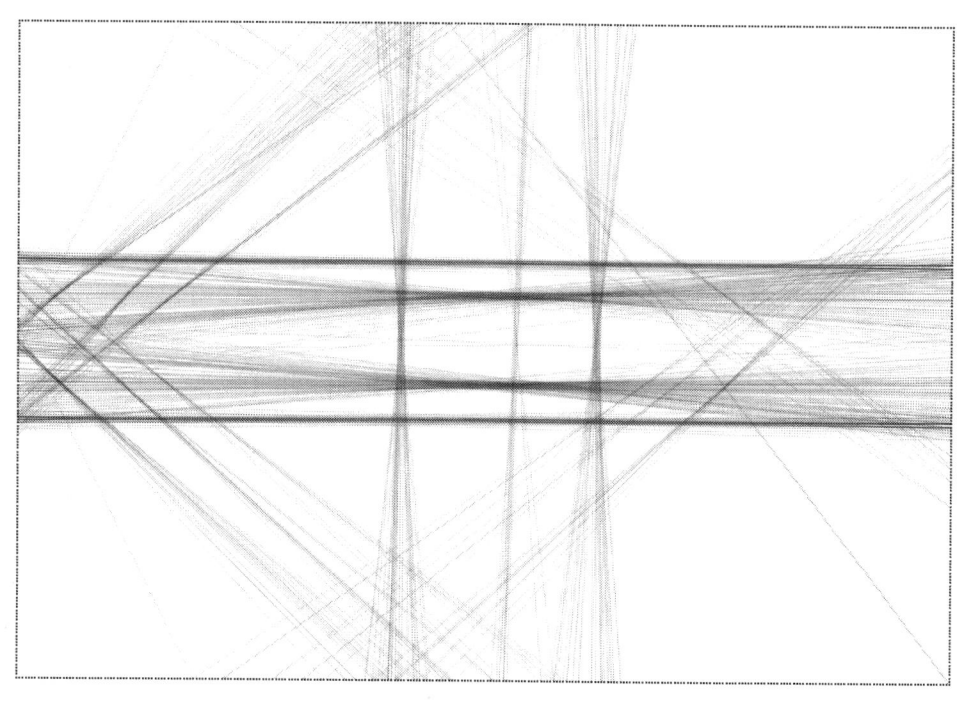

Chapter 7

ROUND 1

SPOILER ALERT...I WAS NOT ready for this shitshow. Here is how I experienced the "miracle" of IVF.

We decided to start our IVF journey in January 2021. *Journey*—what a stupid word, but it is the word that is used in IVF circles. It definitely did not feel like a journey while we were on it. It felt more like the most horrible road trip ever, with stops at Hope City, Devastation Falls, and Trauma Town on a constant loop. Sure, there were other "passengers" who were on this journey, but it did not make it any better. It still sucked.

We were due to start our injections in mid-January 2021. As nervous as I was, I was also excited. We were going to have a baby. I really want to laugh at my younger self, but simultaneously I want to be her. So naive and full of hope. I am no longer that person. I see the world through different eyes, and I know that life is cruel and there is nothing you can do to change that.

When we first started our journey, I was not yet aware of what it actually entailed emotionally. I was blissfully unaware of what was waiting on me. I knew my privacy was going to invaded on many levels during the IVF cycle, and the word *dignity* would only be one that appeared in a dictionary. I did not care about that. It was a small price to pay for having a baby. I do, however, wish I was more prepared for the emotional aspect.

I had to go on the contraceptive pill for a couple of weeks to induce a withdrawal bleed, which I have come to learn is not the same as an actual period. I emailed the nurse on the first day of my period and she told me to go for a blood test—the first of many.

Sitting at my desk at work that morning, I waited for the nurse to let me know if it was all good. It came, and so did a bunch of instructions as to when I had to do the injections. I felt like I could not breathe. I could feel the emotions welling up inside of me. I could not control them. Half-walking, half-running to the bathroom, I started crying. The fear and uncertainty became too much. I was scared—scared of the needles, scared of IVF not working, scared of what people would think, you know, the shame of it all. The shame I felt was 110% unjustified, yet I could not help feeling it.

I let my husband know that we needed to start stabbing me with needles that night. By that night, I had decided that I would not be able to inject myself. Not by a long shot, pun intended. My husband was going to have to do it. It was the least he could do. Six pm was injection time. It ticked closer. He started preparing the first injection, which was a follicle stimulating hormone injection. Like a real pro, he watched a YouTube video to make sure he did it right, and he was ready to inject me. I, on the other hand, was not ready for him to inject me.

He hadn't even come near me to try, and I was already crying. I am not talking about a few tears. No, I was sobbing uncontrollably. You know those ugly sobbing sounds that sometimes escape you when you are really sad? Yep, I had those. All because of one tiny needle. Every time my husband tried to come near me, I burst into tears. To this day I am not sure why I broke down, but it was probably a combination of fear and a whole lot of other emotions.

With a lot of encouragement, I mustered up all the courage I could find, pinched my skin, and closed my eyes. My husband plunged the first needle into my stomach. I hated every second of it and it felt like the injection was lasting forever. When he was finally done, he told me how proud he was of me. With the words "first one done", he lifted his hand up in a high five. I didn't want to high-five him, although I did give him a feeble attempt at one. Although I was proud of myself for getting through the first one, I remembered that I had to do about twenty more where they came from. I get that my husband just wanted to celebrate the small wins, but at that moment, all I wanted to do was cry.

The next day, my husband organised for us to go see some friends. Apparently, we were not going to let IVF ruin our social life—or at least, *he* wasn't. I was completely content hiding from the world during this process. It was just the second night, and I honestly didn't feel like facing people. I resented him for convincing me that it would "be good for me". We had to do the injection at their house. Popping it into the fridge like it was nothing, we chatted away with our friends. They didn't ask many questions. I also don't think they got why we were doing IVF. We were so young; we had plenty of time, right? They just didn't get it. I remember vaguely when my husband tried to explain to a friend that he had no sperm. Innocently, they asked if it would come back if we gave it some time. Their lack of comprehension frustrated me. It was exhausting enough to pretend like my life was not falling apart; I did not have the energy to deal with their stupid questions. I was not mad at them, but more just mad that they didn't get what we were going though. Even during the early stages of IVF, I felt completely alone.

That night, just before 6 pm, we headed up to my friend's room to do the injection. There was no way in hell I was going to do the whole thing in front of them. My husband injected me, sat with me for about two minutes, and left. This did not sit well with me. This whole process was extremely emotional for me, and it felt like all of my emotions were heightened. Him just plunging injections into me and then leaving me there half in tears due to being overwhelmed felt disrespectful and I hated him.

Why did he get to inject me while I had to be the one sitting with the sore stomach and emotions that were all over the place? How was that fair at all? Then he had the audacity to go downstairs and continue playing board games as if my life wasn't falling apart. It was not his fault that I felt the way I did, nor was it his fault that I felt that he acted inappropriately. Looking back, he was just trying to get through it, just as I was. He was just better at hiding the hurt than I was.

My friend, Lily, came upstairs after a while to check on me. She is honestly one of the most empathetic people I have ever met. I just talked my heart out with her for a little bit. She didn't judge. She didn't tell me that I had no right to feel the way I did. She just sat there listening. It is one of the things I appreciated about her. She didn't need to understand what I was going through. She was just there.

The next few days continued in a blur. The only thing I remember is me dreading 6 pm every day, crying, and getting injections. By day 5 of injections, it was time for another blood test and a follicle scan to see if the medication was stimulating my follicles to grow. For those who do not know, follicles are those things that contain eggs. They need to grow to a certain size to ensure that the eggs, if they contain any, are mature. Only mature eggs will be able to be used for fertilisation.

I scooted down on the horrible cold chair, feet in the stirrups, "ready" for the internal ultrasound. I felt so violated, but I just laid there, hoping beyond hope that the medication was doing what it was meant to do. Doctor counted and measured the follicles. He looked a little concerned, but did not say anything except that they were still a little small. I could feel the tears welling up inside me again. All I could think was, *Great. Not only can I not grow follicles by myself, but my body isn't even smart enough to do it when the hormones are supposed to force her to do it..* I should have been kinder to my body, but I didn't care. I hated her for being so utterly useless.

"We need to up your dosage", the doctor said. "We are going to give you the highest dose, and hopefully, your body will respond".

Hopefully! IVF really is the worst—there is no guarantee that your body will do what it is told. You just need to hope and pray until you are blue in the face. Walking out, a tear ran down my face. Gosh, I am amazed at how much I cried during those first few weeks. Hats off to my husband for putting up with that. I always wonder if he got sick of telling me that everything would be okay. Over the course of time, he must have said those same words on repeat about a million times. I honestly got sick of hearing it.

That night we did the higher dose, and we also added a "fun" new injection. This one was supposed to prevent my body from ovulating to allow more follicles to mature. This needle was a lot thicker than the other one. I howled in pain when my husband pushed the thick needle through my skin. I didn't want to do it anymore. I felt like shit. There I went, wanting to give up so early in the process. My husband was supportive, but as I had to endure the physical side effects of the medication, all I could focus on was the injustice of it all and him being able to just carry on like nothing was happening.

The days continued with blood tests and a follicle scans every second day. I was struggling to hold everything together. With work, gym, doctor's appointments, blood tests, chores, and just trying to relax, it was too much. As an added bonus, the hormones were starting to kick in, making me feel physically ill. I was bloated, my pants did not fit because of the bloat, my boobs were super sore, and I was emotional and cranky and crying at the smallest things. I could not walk comfortably. I felt like a duck waddling along. I turned everything into an argument—anything from undone dishes to failing to put clothes in the laundry basket. Like I said, some days I am surprised that we made it.

By my third scan, it seemed like the follicles were doing their thing. Doctor wanted to know how my tummy was feeling. I just told him it was sore but fine. I had more of an internal bruising thing going on. I could not touch my stomach. Even lying on my stomach caused me pain. I was not sleeping, either. I didn't tell him any of this. What would he say? That it is normal. Yeah, right—nothing about this was normal; you could put any poetic spin on it, but it still was not normal, and in no version of any reality was it fine, despite what I said.

I only had a few more days of injections left. I had gotten used to two needles a day, and they were going a bit easier. I was meant to go to egg collection the following week, 11 February 2021.

Nervous did not cover it. I started by letting my work know what was happening, and they were more than happy to agree to me having a few days off. I also had to make sure everything was in order for my husband's operation as well. Somehow, I had become the designated administration lady as well, as if I didn't already have enough on my plate.

My husband was also getting nervous about his procedure. Come on, they were going to cut him open and search through his testicular tissue with a microscope, just like searching for a needle in haystack. I didn't tell him back then, but I appreciated him putting his body through that trauma, as it could not have been easy. I also knew he did it without thinking twice, just as I did my part. We did it for us and for a slight chance for us to have a family.

It was time for my last scan prior to egg collection. I can't remember what day it was. We went in and my follicles looked great. There were a fair number of follicles and doctor was happy enough for us to proceed to egg collection in three days' time. I signed the consent form, and he explained the procedure and also stated that there were obviously no guarantees, just because the clinic had to cover their own behind. I signed. It was not like I could not sign. I was sitting with a body stuffed full of follicles and it felt like I was going to explode.

Later that afternoon, the doctor called. *That's odd*, I thought to myself. *I was not expecting a call.* I picked up the phone. He was his usual friendly self, but I could hear concern in his voice. My blood results came back. My oestrogen levels were low. In other words, we might not get many, if any, mature eggs. I did not understand. I did everything I was told to do. How could this have happened? The doctor explained that we had two options. One, we could proceed to egg collection and not get any mature eggs. Two, we could cancel the cycle and try again next month. I did not know what to do. I could feel my throat close up. Feelings of failure started surfacing again. Logically, I knew it was not my fault, but emotionally, I felt the opposite.

My husband was busy with a meeting (working from home), but I signalled to him that we had to talk, now! I had told the doctor that we would ring him back. My husband got out of his meeting and, with tears streaming down my face, I explained to him what the doctor had told me. He is forever calm in stressful situations, or maybe he took on the role as I was clearly emotionally unstable. He asked me what I wanted to do, because I was obviously the one that had to do the injections again. He could probably see in my eyes that I did not want to cancel the cycle. It had been so hard to do the injections. I was tired and sore. It felt like if I cancelled that it was all for nothing. I had put my body through this process for nothing. I did not want him to see the pain in my face, but I could not keep it in. I broke down. I cried, sobbed, and screamed. It was probably a combination of physical pain and emotional pain. Hating the world, I sat on the couch, hugging a pillow, bawling my eyes out. I was left feeling alone, sad, and embarrassed. I would need to tell my work that I was a failure and cancel my leave. Just the thought of it made me cry even harder.

Despite me feeling like this, my husband felt it was best to cancel the cycle. That way, we at least wouldn't pay the full fee for the IVF cycle and would hopefully have a better chance of success. *Great*, I thought. *No-one cares how Sonja feels, as long as we save money.* I just added being upset with him to the list of emotions I was feeling. How dare he be logical in my time of emotional need. I needed him to be on my side, not play the logic police. I was also mad at the doctor. He had one job, and he couldn't get it right. Most importantly, I was mad at myself for failing. I felt like I had failed a test somehow. I had worked hard and done all the injections, appointments, and dreadful ultrasound scans. I put my whole being into the cycle. Yet I still failed. I hated myself and I hated my body.

My husband called the doctor back, putting him on speaker. The doctor explained everything to him again and asked what we would like to do. I could not get myself to utter those words. My husband did it for me. As soon as he spoke the words "we think we are going to cancel", I broke down again.

For a large part of the afternoon, I remained fixed in position on the couch, hugging a pillow, jumping between crying uncontrollably and just staring out in front of me trying to figure out what I was supposed to do. My husband, on the other hand, just went back to working—how insensitive. I wanted him to join me in my pity party. Sure, it was not helping anyone to sit and cry about it. As I was told when I was younger, "Crying is not going to change anything," but this is how I was dealing with things. I was technically also still on the clock at work, but I just didn't care. I watched email after email pop up on my screen, but I was simply not able to bring myself to do work or even let my job know that I won't be going in for my collection. No, I was just going to sit there, feel sorry for myself, and wait for life to pass me by until I felt better.

Eventually, I plucked up the courage to tell my work that my cycle was cancelled but that I would still like to take one of those days as a "me day". They were surprisingly kind and sympathetic to my situation, which I did not expect but certainly embraced.

I spent the next few days in a deep, dark hole of depression, self-loathing, and yelling at my husband for every little thing. I had so many emotions, I did not know what to do with myself. I was clearly not equipped to deal with failure. Who could blame me? As I said, I had pretty much gone my entire life without any huge failures up until then. At that moment, staring at the wall in front of me, that very white wall, I felt cheated and like this thing that just happened was the worst thing that could ever happen to me. I was wrong.

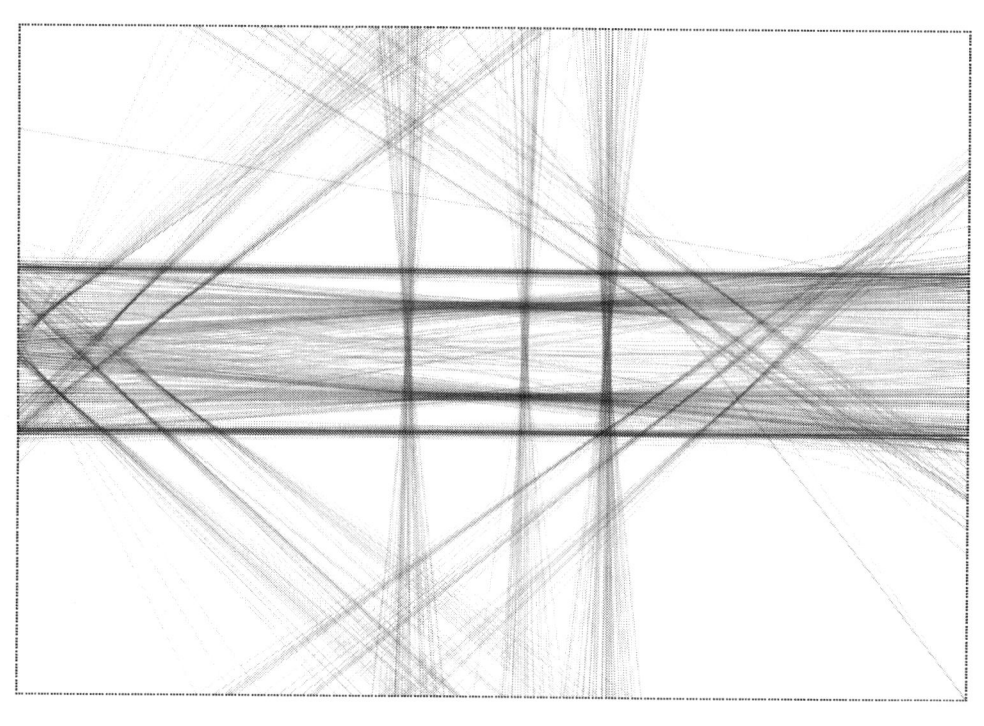

Chapter 8

MY 30ᵀᴴ BIRTHDAY

AFTER A FEW WEEKS of wallowing, feeling sorry for myself, and unpacking my emotional baggage onto my good friend Sam, I started feeling a bit more motivated. Sam is one of my good friends back in South Africa. She is another one of those special people who has sympathy for days and is always happy to lend an ear. I have lost count of how many times I talked to her about the same thing, just going around and round in circles. Not once did she tell me that she was sick of hearing of my struggles. She was and still is always there for me.

My husband decided that we should give it one "normal ovulation" cycle for me to recover and reboot, so to speak. In essence, I needed some time to forget how awful the entire experience was so I could do it again. I needed to remember why I was willing to do it the first time. During our "off" month, I told myself multiple times that I could not do it again and I started to question if I actually wanted to do IVF at all. Now, however, I can readily admit that the only reason I was convincing myself of my incompetence or questioning my motives was because I was scared. I was dead scared of failing again. If I failed, it would just reassert my then opinion that I was a useless failure and an excuse of a "woman". I started to develop body issues when we got our diagnosis, and while going through IVF, it got significantly worse. I was not sure how I would go the second time.

My thirtieth birthday was coming up. Yep, the big three-oh. Just another reminder that I haven't achieved my goals. First kid at thirty. Delusional, I was! It seems laughable now, but when I wrote my ten-year plan, it all seemed so realistic. My sister was pregnant with her third child on her thirtieth birthday. Yet, here I was, childless at age thirty. If we were living in the olden ages, I would have been classified as a spinster. Ironically, my marriage certificate states that my status before I was married was indeed a spinster. Maybe my fate was already sealed and I just did not know it at the time.

As time drew closer, I picked up my provisional IVF plan for the following month and, as I looked at it, the egg collection date struck me immediately: 25 March 2021. One day before my birthday. My mind did some sort of loop-the-loop and illogically deduced that the date must be some sort of sign. Birthdays bring good luck, right? Immediately I felt full of hope that this cycle was going to go great. The fertility gods were probably looking down at me and laughing their arse off at my naivety.

We started our injections again. I somehow expected that it would be easier this second time around; it wasn't my first rodeo. But I was wrong. The second go was no easier than the first. In all honesty, it was harder. Maybe it was because I knew how I would be feeling in a couple of days. Every injection my husband plunged into my stomach killed me a little bit from the inside, but I put on a brave face and tried to live my life.

I tried filling myself with positive thoughts during the two weeks I was injecting myself like a junkie. Oh, how people loved to tell me that if you have positive thoughts, things will happen for you, as if thinking positively is going to make me fertile. Idiots. Despite my personal opinion on the whole "think positive" front, I had positive mantras coming out of my ears, every morning getting a little pop-up on my phone telling me that I was amazing and that "I got this". My husband also loved saying "you got this". He probably didn't really know how to help me and staying positive was his way of contributing to our shitty situation. I, on the other hand, just found it annoying and unhelpful. It was so easy for him to say "you got this" when he was not the one having to go through the physical changes.

At least my follicles were growing amazingly this time around. I was on the highest dose of follicle stimulating hormones, and lo and behold, it was working. They were tracking perfectly. My hope thermometer was filling up. I was even happy to ride the hormonal dragon, pretending every day at work that I didn't want to yell at every second person who asked me how I was.

That simple question could put me on edge. It probably would have been easier if I put a sign somewhere telling them that I was extremely hormonal, about to explode, and that they should just leave me alone. Unfortunately, that is not professional at all. No, I just sat there, smiling, crying on the inside like a champion.

I took my hormones out on my husband, and I wouldn't even have blamed him if he left me. In the early stages, even though I didn't see it back then, IVF placed a huge stress on our marriage. I was trying to hold my shit together while my husband had to endure endless emotional spells, unnecessary arguments, and yelling matches that all boiled down to me saying he didn't know what I was going through. I've said it once and I will say it again: I am not sure how our marriage survived, but I am glad it did.

By the end of week one, I had to see another fertility specialist as my doctor was on leave. I was not happy about this. The main reason was that I would need to spread my legs for yet another random man. I swear I was seeing more action down there than I have ever had in my life, and I hated every moment of it. Sure, they give you a little blue thing to cover up the last bit of dignity you have, but let's face it, they still need to look when they put the ultrasound in. There was only an illusion of dignity and privacy no matter what you think.

The stand-in doctor did, however, deliver some brilliant news. I had more than eighteen good follicles and all were measuring the perfect size to be able to contain a mature egg. I only had to do one more follicle scan in a couple of days and we could go to collection. I was absolutely elated. We were going to go to egg collection this time. For a moment, I even forgot how sore and uncomfortable I was. It was all going to be worth it.

My husband's surgery arrangements were in place. We had organised for Lily to come and pick us up at the hospital, and I had already put in leave at work. Everything seemed to be going well. Doctor B confirmed that everything was looking great and that we could go to egg collection in a few days.

I was to take the trigger injection the following night. The trigger injection is basically the injection that tells your body that it should release the eggs, and then thirty-seven hours later, you have your egg collection procedure. We just needed to confirm my blood work was all good.

My blood work came back, and we once again received a call. My oestrogen was very high, and I was at risk for OHSS: ovarian hyperstimulation syndrome. OHSS is basically an exaggerated response to excess hormones that causes ovaries to swell and become super painful. In some cases, it can be life-threatening, with fluid leaking into your abdomen. We had a plan, though—we were going to put me on a different trigger, and it was going to help me to not overstimulate. I was not convinced, but I had to have faith. My faith had waned a lot through the IVF process at that stage, and I was not sure I would be able to scrape together what was needed, so instead of focusing on myself, I conjured up a new worry that I had pushed down to a deep pit in my brain.

What could that worry be? My husband? Ding ding ding! Being worried about his surgery was the lucky winner. What if they didn't find any sperm during my husband's operation? What then? Do we just use the donor sperm? The thought of having a child with DNA different to that of my husband scared me. Yet the desire to have a family overruled every feeling I might have had. So, down went that worry, back down into the pit where it came from. If I didn't think about it, it didn't exist.

We injected the trigger at exactly the time we were told to do it. It all felt a little bit anti-climactic. I had built it up in my head to be some sort of big moment, but in reality, it was just another injection. It did bring a feeling of relief. *No more injections*, I thought to myself. I got eighteen follicles—that would be plenty of eggs to make embryos. We were set.

The twenty-fifth of March 2021 arrived. We checked my husband into the hospital and then Lily walked with me across the street to check me in. I sat in silence in the waiting room. It is a really odd feeling, sitting in a waiting room with your too-white gown, booties, and a hair net. I sat there watching all the other women, each of us sitting there, praying and hoping by ourselves that we would get our miracle, our rainbow baby.

The anaesthetist came to get me. We had a little chat about what was going to happen. I zoned out while he was speaking, thinking to myself, *I am going to be unconscious, and a bunch of people are going to see me naked and a doctor is going to stick a needle up there, sucking eggs out of my ovaries; it sounds fucking fantastic.* The scientist knocked on the door to let me know that they found some sperm with my husband. I felt unburdened. One fewer thing I had to worry about. The man was a trooper, and it had paid off. Now it was my turn. I had to pluck up my courage, put on my big girl pants, and get some eggs sucked out of me.

Before I got to do this, the doctor came in to chat with me. It felt like I was on a train and, at every station, I had to give my ticket to the train operator confirming that I knew what I was doing and how I was going to get there. It was super annoying. As we spoke, I felt tears welling up in my eyes. I was so, so scared. It was the uncertainty of what they might find in there. Dr B was also going to do a hysteroscopy while he was in there. It was basically just a procedure to check out my uterus, you know, just to make sure nothing was awry. What scared me the most about the procedures was that I was going to be unconscious and not in control. It wasn't that I did not trust my doctor. No, he was great. I just wanted to be able to control the outcome of what was going to happen. The realisation that I couldn't ate me up.

I was asked if I was ready. I nodded my head and we walked into the theatre, having a chat about daily things. There were a lot of people in the theatre. There was my doctor, the anaesthetist, about two or three nurses, and a scientist/embryologist. I was directed to lie on the bed and put my legs in the stirrups. I could feel myself wanting to cry again. It is dreadful having to lie on a bed and place your feet in stirrups while you don't have any underwear on in a room full of people. I did as I was told. *At least I shaved*, I thought. As if the doctors and nurses cared whether I shaved or not. I was just another person heading through the station, but somehow, I thought I was special, like I was the only person who had to go through this, but I wasn't. So many other women were doing exact same thing that day, probably having the same thoughts I had.

Before I went to sleep, the doctor said that he would write the number of eggs they got on my hand for when I woke up. The anaesthetist came and gave me happy gas. You know, because the almost thirty-year-old woman was too scared to have an IV. Everyone's voices faded and it just became a jumble of noises sounding like they were talking over each other but on fast forward, and I heard the sound of the machine. I dozed off. The last thing I heard was a machine almost sounding like I was flatlining as I went into oblivion.

The procedure was not meant to take very long, but it felt like I had been out for ages by the time I woke up. It took me a while to realise where I was. It only took a few seconds for the pain to kick in. It felt like I was being stabbed in the uterus. Almost like period pain, but times ten. It was excruciating. I couldn't find my voice to call the nurse, but somehow, she sensed that I needed her. She looked at me with pity and I was not sure why.

"Did you see your hand? Are you okay?" she asked.

I was confused. I was in pain. What was this woman talking about? I told her I was just in pain and would like something for that. She gave me that pitying smile again and went to get me an analgesic and a heat pack. I was too scared to look at my hand. It was obviously bad otherwise she would not have asked if I was okay. I wanted to look and did not want to look at the same time.

Taking a deep breath, I turned my hand so I could see the top of it. I was shocked. I was confused. I was heartbroken. It was a big fat zero. Zero eggs. I had eighteen follicles and got zero eggs. Devastation did not even begin to cover it. I started crying silently. I was embarrassed. That familiar feeling of failure washing over me yet again. I felt like I was not even worth being called a woman. I could feel tears running down my cheeks, but I did not make a sound.

The nurse came with the meds and heat pack. After taking them, I told her, "I want to go home now." Unfortunately, I had to wait for the doctor, as he wanted to come and see me. I felt numb inside and deeply envious of the woman next to me who was crying because she only got four eggs. If she only knew how lucky she was. The doctor came around and I could see the pity on his face. He told me what I already knew: they got zero eggs. He was just as shocked as I was. He said that it could sometimes happen. It is called empty follicle syndrome, but it could also be that my body did not respond to the trigger. He continued, saying that they only explored one ovary and that they gave me another trigger in theatre. I suddenly had a vague memory of someone asking me for consent and then something being plunged into my stomach. I was not sure if the memory was real or made up and I simply did not care.

My world had just come crashing down. Every single injection I did was for nothing. I got no fucking eggs and it fucking sucked. Why did I have to go through this? What did I do to deserve this? The whole cycle felt like a failure. Sure, we got some sperm from my husband, but what is the use of sperm if we had no eggs? I felt like I somehow failed my husband. I failed to be a wife and a woman. I failed to give him something that he not only yearned for but deserved. He had done his part, and here I was not even remotely doing my part. No, I contributed fuck-all.

Due to them giving me another trigger in theatre, I had the fun "opportunity" to go through the whole process all over again the next day. I was so sore already I didn't even feel physically up to it, but I had to do it. Lily came to pick me up, and as soon as she asked how it went, I had to tell her that the cycle was a dud, that we got zero eggs, and that we would need to do it again the next day. She gave me a hug and it just made me cry even more.

My husband was waiting for me in the car. I was not sure if he had heard the news. He was already in physical pain; now I was just going to lump on the emotional pain. He got out of the car and gave me a hug, and I could sense that he already knew. We got in the car, and he held my hand.

While we were heading home, the doctor called, just relaying for a third time what had happened. I wondered in that moment how many times I would be able to hear the words "zero eggs" before I completely lost my shit. I was not far off. He wanted to talk about what sperm to use if we got any eggs the following day and we decided to put him on speaker. It was a hard decision—do we use my husband's sperm (they only got two vials) if we only get one or two eggs, or do we just destroy the eggs, rendering the cycle a complete and utter failure? I did not know what to say or how to respond. I was broken. It also looked like Lily had tears in her eyes. It was an impossible situation to be in.

We ultimately decided that the doctor would call my husband the following day once the eggs were collected and they would make the call. I trusted my husband enough to know that he would make the right call for us. He tried staying positive for the both of us, saying that there was still hope. For me, there was no hope. All I had was the physical pain and bleeding to remind me that I put myself through that trauma for nothing. I felt like I was bleeding on the inside, blood gushing, but no-one was able to see the wounds bleeding.

I just wanted to lie in a dark room under a million blankets and cry until I had nothing more left. We were staying with Lily and her partner as neither I nor my husband were allowed to drive due to having anaesthesia. I was to put on my "everything is fine" mask and join in the conversation at dinnertime. This was the last thing I wanted to do. I just sat at the dinner table eating my lamb burger and wishing I could be anywhere else. No-one talked about what had happened. I guess there was nothing to really say other than it sucks.

I wanted to yell, scream, and throw things. Most of all, I wished my mum was alive. She would have comforted me in the way that mothers know how to. My dad really tried to be there for me when I told him we got no eggs but, once again, there was nothing he could do or say to make the situation any better. This was our battle and we had to face it. The heartbreak was too much for me to endure and the prospect of having to go through it again the following day was just too much.

I didn't even feel excited for my birthday the next day. I was not excited for the gifts I might receive or the phone calls I was going to take. They were all just painful reminders of how many times I would need to lie to people—"I am good, thank you, how about you?"—the accepted social response to when someone wants to know how you are. The thing is, people rarely want to know how you are. They just ask while walking, most of them not really giving a flying fuck about how you are really doing. They are just doing it because social norm dictates it. It is also really hard to be vulnerable around people who simply do not get it.

The next morning, I woke up feeling dead inside. I had barely slept that night. All I did was cry and worry on a constant loop. I was exhausted. It was like watching a never-ending rerun of the previous day without any ads. Lying there, I did not even feel like getting up. I just felt awful—not birthday-y at all.

Lily, bless her heart, decorated their dining room with the 3-0 balloons and other decorations and even made us some bacon-and-eggs breakfast. I honestly did not feel like eating, although I did. There was no need to insult anyone and, besides, she was trying to make it better somehow, and I did appreciate it. It was one of the sweetest things a person has done for me. That morning, my dad also called. It was more of a "good luck" call than a "happy birthday" call. The thing is, I had already admitted defeat (or so I thought). My husband said that I should hope for the best but prepare for the worst. How did he even expect me to do that? My dad also had a similar view, because there was not really much we could do at that point in time anyway. No-one seemed to understand or even care how I was feeling at that stage.

Riddled with guilt, grief, and sadness, we made our way to the hospital. Everything seemed to pass in a blur. Everyone, from the admissions lady and anaesthetist to the doctor, scientists, and nurses, looked at me with pity. I don't even blame them, as I am pretty sure I looked morbid. The upbeat anaesthetist wished me happy birthday and said that it might bring good luck. Yeah, right, buddy—because luck is why I am having two egg-collection procedures on consecutive days.

The doctor decided to do a scan before they put me under. I felt so self-conscious lying there awake, legs apart, strangers watching, while the doctors pushed the ultrasound up my hoo-ha. *Classy*, I thought to myself. *Congratulations, Sonja. For your thirtieth birthday, you are blessed with failure, embarrassment, guilt, and invasion of privacy. Happy fucking birthday to me.*

As I went under, I was praying like I have never prayed before in my life. I was not bargaining yet—that came way later—but I was praying like my life depended on it. However, all the prayer in the world was not going to change anything. Unfortunately, one thing that IVF took from me is my faith—my faith that if you are a good Christian person, you will be blessed. It was simply not true. I realised it when I woke up in the recovery room in extreme pain and looking down to my hand. This time a number one was written on it. I was disappointed but there was a glimmer of hope. You read so many stories of people who got only one egg that turned into an embryo and they ended up with a pregnancy and live birth. Maybe this was one of those times.

I texted my husband the number and he texted me back a little heart emoji. It felt like he was right there with me even though he was not. Stupid COVID, making things harder than it had to be. He texted me that it was going to be okay, and I decided that, if he had a little bit of hope, I should too.

I got down from that cloud very quickly. The doctor came to my bed, sat down, and held my hand tightly. I have honestly never met a more compassionate doctor in my life. He told me in the gentlest way that he could that, although they did find one egg, it was not mature and that they could not use it. I broke down. Tears flowed from every sense of my being. It felt like my heart broke into a million tiny little pieces. The doctor just sat there with me, holding my hand and not saying anything. He told me to take some time and we could talk later about where we wanted to go from there. They froze the two vials of my husband's sperm.

My husband and Lily came to pick me up. Already knowing the news, my husband gave me a weak smile and held my hand during the car ride. No-one had anything to say. I was crushed. What did I do to deserve this? Was I being punished? The questions just kept coming and each answer was more elusive than the last.

I spent the rest of my day telling people that I had a good birthday and that I appreciated the well wishes. What I actually wanted to tell them was that it was the worst birthday that I had ever had. That night, we had some chocolate cake and rocky road treats as part of my birthday celebrations. We even took a photo of me and my husband. I have kept the photo over the years. I look horrible in the picture—my eyes are swollen, I have no make-up on, and my hair look like I just woke up. I feel like that particular photo is a reminder that, even though things are absolutely horrible in life, you need to find little things to celebrate. I did not feel like that at that stage, but now I am happy that we did take the photo.

The next day, my husband and I were off to our own house again, leaving our friends' home a little less hopeful and a little more broken, but at least we still had each other.

The morning we left their house, I was terribly upset, although I did not show it, or maybe I did; I can't remember. Why, you ask? How could I be so ungrateful towards friends who let me stay at their place for two days and drove me to and from the hospital? The thing is, the day after my birthday, 27 March 2021, was the baby shower of another friend of ours. I did not care that we were not invited, as I honestly did not want to go. I would just have had a breakdown and ruined all the good vibes. I was just mad at them celebrating someone else's baby, someone else's fertility. How could they go there and be happy and excited for someone else having a baby while knowing that I had just failed miserably in not only having a baby but making eggs at all. How inconsiderate could they be? I knew these thoughts were irrational, and I knew that the hate I was harbouring was not toward them or even towards our pregnant friend. No, the hate that I had, and sometimes still have, is towards the injustice of it all. Why did some people get to be blessed and have baby showers and be excited about bringing a new life into this world and I was not allowed to have any of that? It felt like they were insensitively rubbing fertility in my face. I hated every fertile person at that point.

To sum up, I did not get to have a great birthday, a good egg collection, or the hope of any baby at all. No, I was stuck with having nothing, and that concluded the worst birthday of my life, folks. However, this cycle was far from over; it was a gift that kept giving in the most unfortunate way.

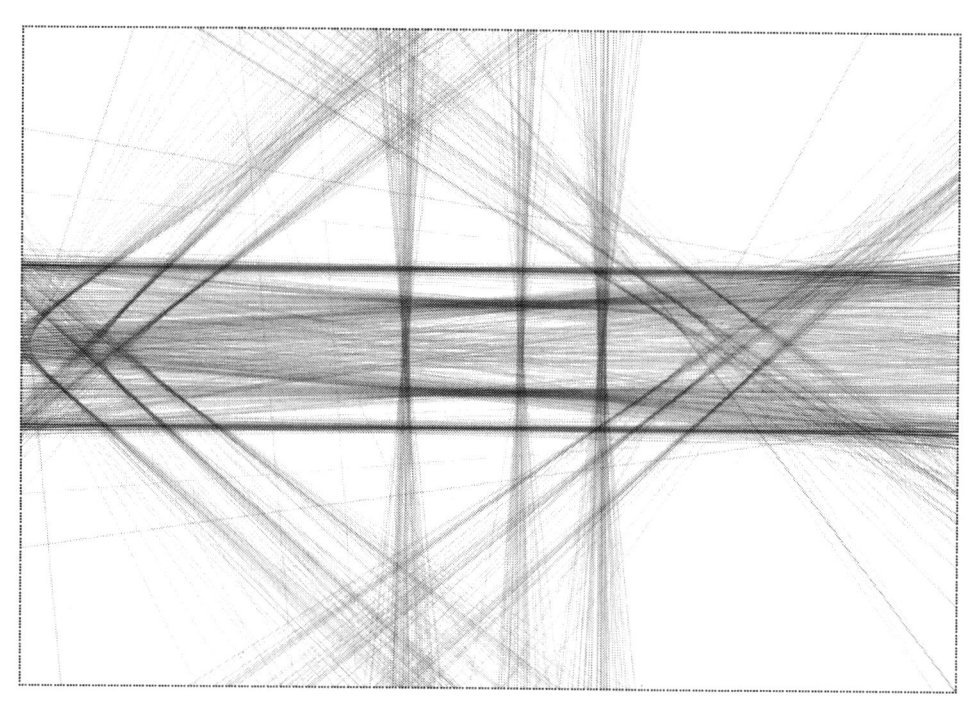

Chapter 9

IVF – THE 'GIFT' THAT DID NOT STOP GIVING

THE NEXT FEW DAYS were spent crying and researching, trying to find answers as to why I had no eggs retrieved. I still could not wrap my head around it. The stupid internet kept throwing the word "empty follicle syndrome" at me. Typing that into Google basically just got me a few pages saying that it usually happens to older woman or people with a low ovarian reserve. I knew my reserve was low, but was it really that low? I also could not stop thinking about how I failed my husband. How I did not do my part. Even though he didn't once say it or make me feel like I failed him, I made it my personal mission to bring myself down, using myself as a punching bag. I wish I could tell my younger self that she should really not be that hard on herself. Sometimes things just happen without reason or understanding. However, younger me felt compelled in giving herself an emotional beating, and I was nothing but thorough.

The following Monday, I had to work because, unfortunately, life doesn't pause just because you are falling apart. No, adulthood is a sadistic concept where you keep working and put on a brave face because that is just life. Looking back, my work probably would have given me the day off had I asked. I was just too damn stubborn and wanted to pretend I was fine. Pretending was easier than admitting defeat.

I had been feeling "off" the entire day. I couldn't stand up straight without being in extreme pain. Walking two minutes caused me to be out of breath and I was nauseous like you would not believe. Instead of opting to call my specialist or his nurse, I went on the IVF support group page to ask people if feeling this was normal. I mean, it was my first egg collection, maybe feeling like this was the prize you got for putting your body through torture and not getting anything out of it. Like a bonus prize for participation.

All the women told me to go to the emergency room immediately, as it could be OHSS. *Nah,* I thought. *Doctor gave me the other trigger so I would not get OHSS.* My husband asked me if he should take me, and I insisted that I was going to wait it out. Maybe, just maybe it will go away on his own. Spoiler alert! It did not. It wasn't even an hour after I told my husband to wait that I gave in. I really did not want to go to the hospital, but I had no choice. My husband drove me to the closest hospital, which luckily was only about a five-minute drive. He could not go in with me because, you know, COVID. I was taken into the emergency department to wait for a doctor. I have never felt so alone and scared in a long time. I waited and waited, but no-one told me what was happening.

Eventually, a doctor came by to ask me how many follicles I had prior to going into collection and how many eggs were retrieved. I felt ashamed to tell him that, even though I had eighteen follicles, I got zero eggs. He nodded and left. A nurse arrived shortly after, putting an IV in. I have to applaud the nursing staff, though. They were so kind and gentle that, even though I was scared, they made me feel at ease. The next hour passed. It was a blur of white walls, beeping noises, people in masks, and travelling voices. The pain medication was kicking in and eased up my pain with the con of added confusion. My husband kept messaging me about every thirty minutes or so just to check in, but the status report remained "waiting".

After what felt like forever, they told me they were going to send me for an ultrasound to check my ovaries. Finally, something was happening. I met with the person who would be doing my ultrasound. It was a man. *Great,* I thought. *Another man to add to the list of who has seen my hoo-ha.* He looked a bit inexperienced, or maybe it was just because he seemed so young. He looked about in his mid-twenties.

They rolled me into the ultrasound room and, with a lot of difficulty, I got on the bed. First question: "Is there any chance you are pregnant?" He clearly did not read my file. Tears welling up in my eyes, I gave a cold no. Second question: "When was your last period?" For fuck's sake, is this guy for real?! Did he buy his degree at AskIrrelevantQuestions.com? A tear slipped down my cheek and my voice quavered as I had to explain to him that I don't ovulate by myself. He wrote it down. By this time, I had lost my temper, asking him if we could just get on with it. He nodded, and then he handed me the ultrasound wand because, for some reason, he could not put it in himself.

He proceeded to look at my ovaries, pushing so hard it felt like my ovaries were going to pop any minute from the pressure. I could see on the screen that all my follicles were still there, and they were huge. He took the ultrasound wand out. You know, because taking it out himself is so much different than putting it in himself. I was rolled back to the emergency department. It was almost 11 pm when I was told that it was OHSS and that I would need to be admitted.

My husband had brought me a few things in the meantime, and they were all taken up to my room. Luckily, a single room. Sitting in the bed, I hated everyone and everything and I was mad. Mad at the world, mad at God for making this happen to me; just mad. I was probably feeling a whole lot of other emotions, but I chose to focus on the anger rather than the sadness.

Just before 12 pm, a nurse came in and gave me the rundown of things. I would need to be weighed every morning and evening to check my water retention because, you know, it is every woman's dream to get on a scale twice daily. The doctor called around 12:30 pm to check up on me and to see if I was okay. Bless his heart. There are many doctors in it for the money, but I firmly believe to this day that he is not one of them. He confirmed a diagnosis of OHSS and also told me how sorry he was that this happened. It was like a double whammy. No eggs and OHSS. I guess there were far worse things in the world, but it certainly did not feel like it.

The following morning, I got up to go to the bathroom. Turning on the light, I was met by my own reflection. I had bags under my red and swollen eyes. Tear stains clear on my cheeks. Looking at myself, I wondered if this was going to be the rest of my life. Just trying and failing on a constant loop. I stared at myself and, for some reason, the tears came streaming again. I was not sure how my body produced all the tears, because I thought for sure that I was dried up by this stage. I think just seeing yourself so broken makes you sad. All I wanted was to be held tightly by my husband, or just anyone, but all I had to hug was the white hospital pillow, because I was not allowed to see my husband. I could feel the depression was coming out to play and soon.

I called my work from the hospital bed and, with all the professionalism I could muster, I told them that my procedure had some complications and that I would be off work for a couple of days. It ended up being an entire week. My work was once again sympathetic to my circumstances and did not bat an eye.

The week in hospital was good in its own way. It gave me time to not only rest up but to think and grieve. I decided that if my husband was okay with it, I would like to give it another go. They do say three rounds is usually what it takes. Plus, we have already had the two worst outcomes, so there could be no harm in trying.

I was discharged on the Thursday and was met by a bunch of flowers from work. They told me they were from the team but that no-one knew the specifics of what happened. I appreciated the notion, as I did not want everyone to know the ins and outs of my fertility struggles at that stage. As time passed, I did become a bit more open.

I took the rest of the week off to recuperate and to set an appointment with the doctor. I hoped that he had a plan, because what we had tried so far clearly did not work. It became clear to me that our fertility issues were not as simple as we thought. It was no longer a case that it was just my husband with fertility issues. No, there was something wrong with me, too. We just did not know what or why.

We had our next appointment in a couple of weeks, and I took the time to reboot again. Like I said earlier, time to forget and shove everything that happened down so I could "move on".

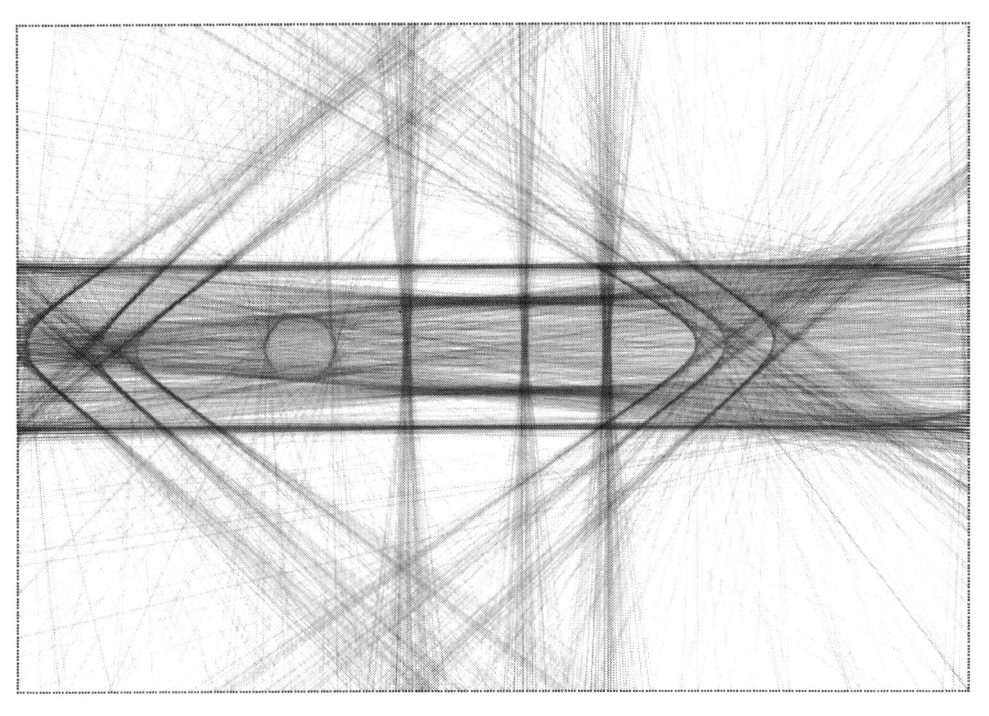

Chapter 10

THIRD TIME'S THE CHARM?

DESPITE HAVING OUR NEXT appointment in a couple of weeks, we decided to take a breather. My body (and mind) needed some time to heal from the traumatic experience. We told the doctor that we wanted to take some time off; not a whole lot, you know, because we don't have much time—my biological clock was kicking down like a bomb getting ready to explode. We landed on a two-month break and decided to have another round in July.

It took a few weeks, but after a while, I started to feel a little normal again, being able to go out and not worry about injection times or any other fertility things. It was like being on a vacation but not. You see, after our second failed egg collection, something happened.

Everything related to babies made me want to weep for weeks. I avoided walking in the baby clothes department, even more than I had before. Oh, how I missed the days of pointing out cute baby clothes to my husband and him smiling and "running away". It was no fun looking at things that you might never be able to have. Even fictional pregnancies started to hurt. I remember re-watching an episode of *The Big Bang Theory* where Bernadette wanted to tell Howard that she was pregnant and all of a sudden I am crying because, you know, why do they get to have it so easy? Fuck them and their fictional lives.

So, even if I was moving on, I was also not moving on. I couldn't. I was just stuck on this hamster wheel of not being able to conceive, my mind running and running in circles trying to find solutions and reasons and only occasionally for a brief moment taking a breather to forget. The resting moments never lasted long. My moments of normalcy were always interrupted by a small thing that would trigger my thoughts and feelings.

It hurt so fucking badly. Even scrolling through social media and seeing a post of someone announcing their pregnancy or doing a gender reveal cut me deeply, and to this day, it still does. I hated these women and their pregnancy announcements. We were not super close, and I did not want any harm to come to them or their child, but boy, did I hate them. I hated that they were fertile, and I hated that they could announce a pregnancy and I couldn't. I just hated them. They did not deserve to be silently hated; it wasn't their fault, and for all I knew, they had also struggled with infertility and got their miracle baby. However, even that did not mitigate my hate. No. I was set on feeling all the anger. I guess in the great span of things, it's easier to hate than to hurt.

I also felt like I was withdrawing socially. I am already an extremely introverted person and people don't always get me, but I withdrew even more. The main reason was that we were at an age where women started talking about starting a family. I was always one of those women, joining in on the conversation about our make-believe families and futures.

On our way to a girls' night, I confided in one of my friends that I really hoped people were not going to talk about babies, as it was really hard for me. I was seeking support but did not get it. All she had to offer was that women talk about these things and I just basically needed to deal with it. Deep down I knew it was true, but it is hard to explain to someone that it is not so easy to deal with. It is hard to explain how participating in conversation about babies kills you on the inside when you know it might never be in the cards for you. It is even harder to hold your shit together and not break into a million pieces when someone asks you when you and your husband are going to start a family. It is interesting how people use "when" and not "if". As if there is nothing in the world that could cause you not to be able to have a child or if having a child is the only real goal in life.

While at the girls' night, we were all sitting in the living room having a chat and suddenly the conversation of babies came up. I zoned out for some of the conversation, but as it continued, I felt my throat tightening and tears welling in my eyes. I swallowed, blinking back the tears. "We" were talking about what language we would raise our children in when we had them. Some of us were bilingual (Afrikaans and English), so it was probably a fair question. I sat there screaming everything I wanted to tell them inside my head. I wanted to tell them that they shouldn't just assume someone can have kids. I wanted to tell them that there was someone in the room who was struggling and would rather not talk about something she might never get to decide. I wished I could have said all of those things, but instead, I just sat there in silence, not participating in the conversation but internally having a breakdown. I was not close enough to these women to have an emotional breakdown due to my infertility, and I was certainly not going to be known as the person who ruined girls' night.

One of the girls obviously wanted to include me in the conversation although I was perfectly happy to be a silent observer. The question came: "What about you, Sonja? Will you raise your kids Afrikaans, English, or both?" I wanted to come straight out and tell her that I didn't know if we would be able to have kids as we were struggling with infertility. Instead, like a coward, I said, "I don't know; probably both."

When I got back home, I had a good cry over what was, for me, not the greatest of nights, and I once again moved on. I sometimes wonder how many times one can move on before you just break. I have "moved on" and "let it go" many times over the years, but it never took long for me to have another breakdown. It is probably because I never really moved on, as I didn't give myself the room and kindness to express what I was really feeling. I sometimes wish I could be one of those women who did not want to have kids; life would have been so much easier. I was not living my best life, and I hated it.

We were set to start injections again in mid-June. I psyched myself up, telling myself that a lot of things are "third time lucky". In all honesty, I was not feeling positive or hopeful at all. Before starting the injections, I unpacked the injections I had done thus far. You know, because I kept them for that photo I would maybe be able to take one day. You know, the iconic one with the heart made out of needles with a little sonogram in the middle. That one. So, I unpacked my needles and counted them.

In a nice round perfect circle lay just over fifty needles. *This was a mistake*, I thought to myself. I broke down again. *I have jabbed myself over fifty times and have nothing to show for it.*

Taking a photo of them as a reminder of what I have already gotten through as motivation for the next round, I packed them away. I found my IVF cycle plan and noticed that it had a new medication on it. All the IVF warriors out there who have used this specific medication knows that it burns like a bitch. It is said to be made of pregnant woman's urine. Isn't that a fun thought when you need to inject yourself with it? You might think that I am kidding, but I am not.

Our time arrived and the usual not-so-forgotten routine sprang into action, like we were never on a break at all. They were not lying about the new injection, though. I howled a little bit the first time I got it. The times after that I kind of started swearing multiple times in a row for the whole duration that the needle was in me. I think it somehow distracted me from the pain and it wasn't a bad outlet for emotions, either. Sometimes, I wondered what the neighbours thought, as I was pretty sure they could hear me cursing and, on occasion, howling in pain, depending on where I was at that particular moment. Injections tend to hurt more when you are already blue and bruised, yet you persevere.

To my disappointment, fewer follicles were growing this cycle, but they were growing evenly. As I decided to try and be more positive, I stayed focused on that, for the most part. A little part of me always remained scared that we would fail for a third time.

This time around, I told fewer people that we were doing a cycle. Telling fewer people means disappointing fewer people. It also meant fewer people feeling sorry for you. I could stand many things during our time doing infertility treatments, but one of them I could not was stares of pity. The other thing I could not stand was people telling me that they knew someone who struggled to have kids and they did IVF once and it worked, or people telling me to just relax and it would happen. It's like, WTF? Do these people possess a brain? Relaxing is not going to give my husband sperm and it is not going to increase my ovarian reserve substantially, and just because you know one person who did IVF that does not make you an expert on fertility treatments.

Unfortunately, when dealing with infertility, you deal with a lot of uneducated people who are just trying to help. Fortunately, you also get to talk to women in similar situations. The women who are able to joke about the worst parts of fertility treatments because, if you don't laugh about the indignity of it all, you will cry an ocean.

Egg collection rolled around. For the first time, my oestrogen levels were perfect. I felt good. Yes, I did cry again when the doctor and anaesthetist came to chat with me. The worst is when the anaesthetist remembers you and says, "Didn't I see you just a few months ago?" and you are just sitting there staring at the floor as if it is the most interesting thing in the entire room. Jumping up on theatre bed, I no longer cared about who would see my hoo-ha. I just lay there patiently waiting to have my nap and hoping beyond hope that this time would be different. I also shot up a prayer, just in case.

Waking up the third time around was less painful, but I was also way more scared to look at my hand. I must have lain there for about fifteen minutes before I had to courage to look at my hand. I could not believe it; we got three eggs. I know three doesn't sound like a very good number, and for many, it is not. For us, on the other hand, three was great. Three is way better than the zero we had before. It meant we had a chance to make embryos. Achievement unlocked. We had gotten to the next stage.

I took a photo of my hand and sent it to my husband. He replied with a little heart, and I am pretty sure he felt the same kind of relief I did. Now we had to wait to hear if any of my eggs fertilised. I swear it was the most gruelling twenty-four hours of my life. I had taken the day off work after egg collection and had taken a walk.

I love walking along the Brisbane River; it brings me peace. As I was walking, my phone rang. Recognising the number, I immediately answered. I am almost sure that I stopped breathing while I waited for the person on the other end to talk. Two of our eggs fertilised normally and one had only partially fertilised, but we had a chance. They were also able to use my husband's sperm—bonus! I immediately called my husband and was greeted with a tight hug, one filled with relief and hope, when I got home. This was, however, short-lived. The day after we got the call, the clinic called and said that the doctor would like to do a day three transfer instead of a day five. Apparently, the one that partially fertilised did not make it, and of the other two, only one was looking good. The doctor decided that the embryo would have a better chance inside me than out.

This was uncharted territory for me. I put in leave from work and the next day, with a full bladder, headed to the day hospital for transfer. Time ticked by slowly—tick, tick, tick. It was as if I could hear every second go by. I was starting to wonder if something had gone wrong. Did the embryo not make it? Is there anything to transfer? I found it a bit inconsiderate to let me sit and worry there. They could have just called and said, "Hey, chill out; we got your embryo," but no, I had to sit in gruelling silence for almost two hours. The doctor finally called and said that we had a good embryo. It was as if I was holding my breath for the past two hours and could finally let go. After that, I waited about another ten minutes for the doctor to come and get me.

I went into the room. I felt anxious yet excited, my heart racing. They did not give me a picture of the embryo, and I was a little disappointed. Getting up on the bed, I spread my legs once again, feelings of shame and embarrassment only vaguely present. The embryologist quickly explained that the embryo they were putting back now was a champion, but they would watch the other one overnight. I feel that they sometimes embellish how good an embryo actually is just to instil a little hope. I am not going to lie. It worked. I got to see how a little blib was pushed into my uterus. It was barely noticeable to the naked eye, but it was magic. It was a bit of a shame that my husband could not share in the experience.

The doctor had to take a good few minutes to convince me that the embryo was not going to fall out and that I could just carry on as usual. I had this fear that I would wee or sneeze it out; ridiculous, I know. Walking out, he gave me a blood test form for a pregnancy test to take in ten days. I started thinking how funny it would be to tell people that another man got me pregnant while my husband waited in the other room. Taken out of context it might sound horrible and not a laughing matter, but I preferred to see the humour in it.

I had to start taking progesterone now to make my uterine lining a little more attractive for our little blob. It was absolutely horrible and probably the closest thing I would ever feel to pregnancy. The progesterone made me nauseous, bloated, and cranky, my breasts were super sore, and I have never been more fatigued in my life. What was worse was I kept feeling little twinges and cramps.

Not knowing what was happening in my body started to put me on edge. I started googling and searching my IVF support groups for posts. There would be someone who said they felt a twinge on the left side just below their hip and they ended up becoming pregnant or they had cramps that felt like their period or sore breasts and they had a positive pregnancy test. I knew it was too early to test and the nurses had advised against it, but it was too hard not knowing. I felt like what I imagined being pregnant would feel like, but did it mean I was pregnant? I really wanted to stay in this world where I was PUPO (pregnant until proven otherwise).

I took a couple of days off work watching movies and relaxing with intermittent periods of panic attacks wondering whether I was doing something I should not be doing. I was putting so much pressure on myself, and it was causing my anxiety and stress to become heightened. I became super sensitive, anxious, and as my husband would put it, a little whiny. It was becoming remarkably difficult to recognise myself. Sure, I was a sensitive soul before, but this was a whole other level. The fact that I put the gym aside for the two-week wait did not help at all. I was also stressing that I was working too hard at work. I was only an admin assistant but prided myself on being the best I could be. This caused me to be more stressed than was actually necessary. I feel like I could have done so many things differently back then. Maybe just worry less in general, you know?

I didn't like admitting it, but whether I worried about it or not was not going to determine if the embryo stuck or not. It was out of my control and this control freak's worst nightmare.

It was also a vicious cycle. I was burying myself under work to forget the pressure I was under to "make" the embryo stick but this, in turn, created a pressure of its own. I was so stupid but could not see the madness in my methods.

About seven days post-transfer, I took a pregnancy test. It is a difficult emotion to describe. It is a combination of excitement, anticipation, hope, and dread all mixed together. It is the ultimate recipe for disaster if you add to little or too much of one of the ingredients. In my case, I added too much hope and excitement and forgot to add the caution. I peed on the stick and waited the two minutes. I started at the stick while it did is thing. My heart dropped into my stomach as each second passed. Once again, as all those times before, I was staring at a single pink line. I did not want to upset my husband so decided to bury the test deep in the trash and try again the next day. It might have just been a little too early, I convinced myself.

The next day, another test, another single pink line. For a fleeting second, I thought I saw a faint second line, but it vanished just as quickly as it appeared. I was clearly losing my mind. Once again, I decided not to tell my husband. I was starting to get worried. I was having some period-like cramps, but denial was easier than admitting defeat, so I convinced myself it was just the progesterone.

The next day, I woke up early to take another sneaky test. Why I continued doing this to myself is beyond me. As I wiped, I noticed blood. I broke down in silent tears. Seeing the single line for a third day in row did not make the situation any better. Instead of admitting to myself, I searched the IVF group for posts of people who bled and was still pregnant or who had a negative pregnancy test but positive bloods. I mean, bloods were still an entire day away; let's not jump to conclusions. Luckily for me, and also because you will always find the answer you are looking for if you search hard enough, I found posts of woman who had bled and had negative tests but positive bloods. I was in the clear, I thought to myself; there was still hope.

This time, I opted to tell my husband that I took a test and it was negative. He looked disappointed as he got ready for work. He headed off and I logged in to work. I was working from home; thank goodness for that. I went to the bathroom again around 10 am, and then there was more blood than I thought was "normal". I called the nurse and told her I thought it was my period. Instead of saying, "Stop the progesterone," she said I should go for the pregnancy test right away.

What is one of the most soul-crushing things you have ever had to do? For me, it was going to do a pregnancy test while having my period, just to confirm that I was not pregnant. To make things worse, there was a pregnant lady in the waiting room of the pathology department yelling at her kid. I had my bloods done and headed home. I wished my husband was there, but he was still at work. I don't really know why he didn't come back as soon as I told him the news. Maybe because he thought that it would not change anything or that he could not do anything to make it better. A few hours later, the nurse rang just to confirm, once again, that indeed my HCG levels were zero. I was not pregnant. Another nurse called me a bit later again to say what I had already been told twice and she said that there were steps I could take to address my emotional well-being. If they were knowledgeable at all, they would know telling a person twice in one day that they are not pregnant when they really hoped they were is not the way to go about so-called emotional well-being.

I thought the zero-egg cycle was the worst I could ever feel, but I was wrong. This was worse. Failed implantation is worse. I felt like I let my husband down. I was also mad at him for not being there. I did a recap of my memories trying to find something I did wrong to explain it. Maybe that one time a slipped on the stairs caused it to fail. Maybe I walked too much, or maybe I should not have eaten that fish. The fact of the matter is that there simply was no specific reason they could pinpoint that led up to that moment. It was simply a case of "it is what is". I am pretty sure it was not God's plan, because that would be a terrible plan to let someone suffer like this. There was no reason. I just wasn't pregnant, and I had to accept it.

That night, doctor called to offer his sympathy and said that often the first one does not work. I knew this was statistically true, but hard facts never have and never will make me feel better. We needed time to process our feelings, or at least, I did, and then we would decide on a path forward. I already knew the path, though: I wanted to try again. The thing is, and I forgot to mention it, that none of our other embryos had made it. We had to do another egg-collection round. Injections a fourth time around.

System reboot activated. I started to wonder how many times I would be able to do this. I was sure at that stage that I had not yet reached my limit. I would try again, because what if the next cycle was the one that worked? What if the next cycle was the one to bring me a child?

Before I conclude this chapter, I would like to add the following analogy to my above statement. I can't remember the author, but kudos to them for slamming the hammer on the nail. They said that IVF treatment is like being in an abusive relationship. At first, when you meet, everything is wonderful, and there are a few bumps, but you manage to live with them (injections), a few weeks go by and they start showing their real colours (poor follicle growth, poor egg numbers, poor fertilisation, embryos dying and failed implantation). Then they promise you that they will be better; things will be different if you just gave it another shot (this is a large part of self-convincing and an element of hope before you start a new cycle).

I did not realise it at the time, but I was in an abusive relationship with IVF. I had an addiction to hope where there was only a slight glimmer of it, but I was not yet ready to admit that to myself.

No, we would go on to do another cycle, because there is promise that the next time will be different.

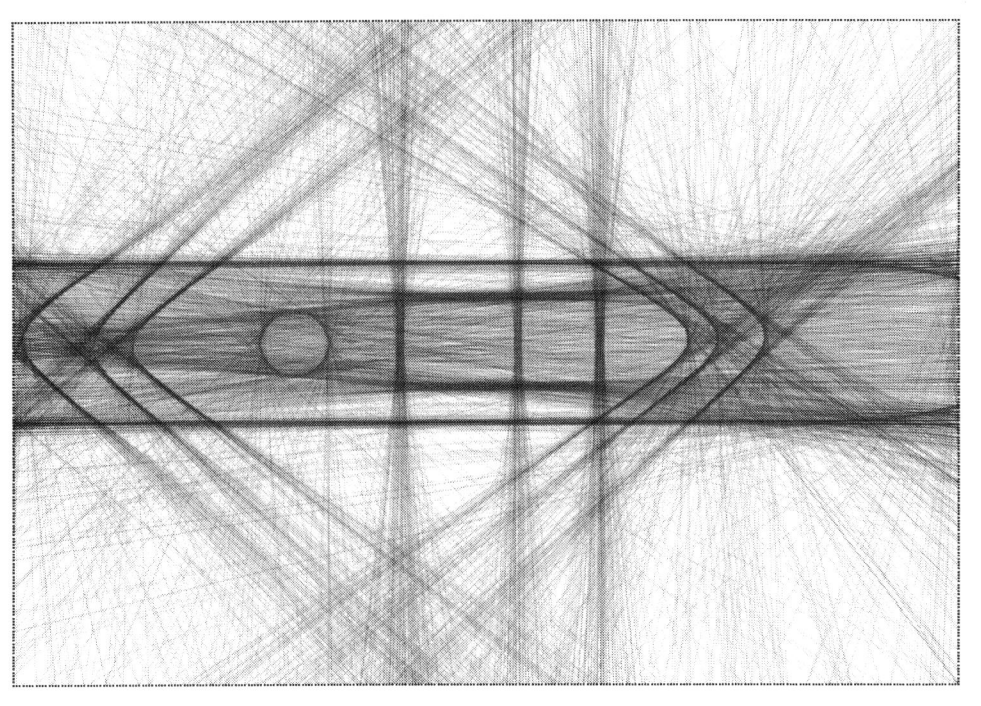

Chapter 11

DÉJÀ VU

SEPTEMBER WAS IN THE air; the flowers were blossoming, and we had just gone through about another two-month break. I felt good, and we were ready to start another round of IVF, the trauma of the previous cycles already tucked away deep in the "let's not think about it" section of my mind.

We went camping for Lily's thirtieth birthday. I am not really the happy camper type, but I make exceptions. My husband and I had a good trip down to the campground and I was happy and just in an overall good mood. Nothing could change that. Haha. Wow, I was getting good at being wrong. It felt like every time I felt good, something fertility-related had to come and bulldoze over what I had just built, even if it was just momentarily.

I was sitting with our friends under the gazebo when I heard the dreaded word "pregnant" topped with "we weren't really expecting it". It felt like I was punched in the gut. The all-too-familiar feeling of tears welling up returned, and once again, I blinked them away. I didn't really stay for the rest of the conversation, but I am pretty sure she said that they were not even trying. I was livid. How dare she get pregnant "without even trying"? I hated her. Feelings of jealously followed by guilt ensued, because I was jealous and mad at the woman who was only trying to share her joy. She wasn't even far along, and it astounded me that someone could announce a pregnancy without a glimmer of fear that she might not carry to term. No, in her world, everything just magically went according to plan.

For the remainder of the weekend, every time I looked at her, all I could think of was the fact that she was pregnant and I was not. She was going to be a mother and have the life that I was supposed to have. What did she do to deserve that, and what did I do to not deserve it? Was she a better person than me? I highly doubted that one of us was better than the other, but it surely didn't feel this way.

It didn't really help that during the weekend there were a bunch of conversations around the topic. People started talking about babies and I opened up to a fellow friend who I knew have also been struggling. However, they never embarked on IVF. I told her and her husband that it was hard to try and try and try with nothing happening. They were always so positive that the next round would work. People do love filling you with false positivity, and I don't blame them. What else is there to say other than "I hope it works next time" or "Don't give up hope; your time will come"? They were doing what any good friends would do; they were trying to be supportive. The relentless positivity was not actually making me feel better. It started feeling like everyone I talked to was on a record and it just kept playing on repeat, saying the same thing over and over again. My positivity was waning. I think it was around this cycle that it started dawning on me that it might not ever happen.

They say that it takes three cycles to get a child. Here we are on cycle number four with nothing. Sure, our first one was cancelled, but I just didn't care anymore. Some days, I just wanted it to be all over so I could live my life, but then I had a fleeting moment where I would imagine my life without children and I just couldn't.

Another friend of ours overheard that we were doing infertility treatments. I confirmed this and, when he asked how many we had done, I told him we were about to start cycle number four. He continued to tell me that he and his wife were worried because the doctors told them they would struggle and will likely need IVF as they were older. My interest was piqued, and I asked the stupid question if they had gone through IVF. His answer disappointed me. He said no. It only took a few months and they were pregnant. He said they "were lucky".

It felt like everyone around me was lucky except for me. They had a beautiful daughter, and I just wanted someone to tell me they did IVF and it actually worked despite doctors telling them that it might be hard. I got the opposite of what I was looking for. I just wanted to cry, but as we were with our friends at a birthday, I had to suck it up. It is, after all, the "adult thing" to do.

The rest of the weekend was quite uneventful, but I found myself withdrawing from our friends more and more. I just couldn't be in the company of people with babies or talking about babies. To this day, I find it a bit hard, and I prefer to steer clear of such conversations and have an escape route if it gets too much—a place where I can go to take a breather. I have done this many times during our journey: fixed up my make-up and gone out pretending that nothing happened, although I have gotten better with dealing as time passed.

After the less-than-fun weekend, I had one more week of "normal". I put that in quotations because, even though we were not doing injections, I was constantly thinking about it and dreaming about it, constantly occupied with what I could do "better" this cycle. I was feeling a little bit more optimistic, though. We decided to try different injections. I was ready.

We went through all the motions: injections, scans, bloods. It was like I was on a repeat of our previous cycle. I also had exactly the same number of follicles growing. It made me fearful that the current cycle would have the same outcome as the last cycle, but I tried my best to ignore the feeling of impending doom.

Egg collection was creeping closer. Aside from the swearing every time I got an injection, I only had one or two meltdowns, not counting the time I broke down in tears because we were out of mayonnaise. That must have been one of my lowest points, but what is a woman to do? You win some battles or you lose them, even if they are just with yourself.

As expected, I experienced déjà vu after egg collection. Opening my eyes in recovery, I looked down at my hand. In black ink on my right hand stood the number three. I was disappointed. I should have known by then not to be too optimistic and to leave room for disappointment, yet every time I fell into the trap of promised rainbows and butterflies. I should have realised that, for us, there was no four-leaved clover, rabbit's foot, or leprechaun that would bring me a pot of gold for good luck. Nope, we were shit out of luck, and I had to make the best of what I had. I was not really doing a good job with "making the best of things". Everything just sucked. I wanted to wallow in the suck and be wrapped in a blanket tightly like a burrito and cry. This response, however, was not socially acceptable.

By this fourth cycle, I told even fewer people that we were doing a cycle. I could no longer tolerate their optimism or positive thoughts and prayers. Even worse, I could not stomach having to repeat bad news over and over again, as every time I had to deliver the same bad news, it felt like a part of me died.

Much like the previous cycle, all three eggs were mature. One fertilised great, and the other two, not so much. I was not sure whether it was the sperm or the egg and the doctor couldn't really tell us, either. It was just the luck of the draw. The luck of which we had none.

It was another day three transfer of an embryo that apparently looked great. I took that with a pinch of salt, as they had no other embryos to compare it to, so it was obviously great, as it was the only one standing. *Stop it*, I would tell myself. *All you need is one good one.* I reminded myself of this constantly throughout the two-week wait.

I read that you should manifest, and then your embryo will stick. At this stage, I would need super glue to make it stick. I wondered if that was an option. All I was thinking during the whole week was, *Stick, little embaby, stick.*

Unfortunately, just like the previous cycle, the embryo did not listen. I took a pregnancy test the day before bloods were due and, once again, I got a big fat negative. I started to feel like my uterus was where embryos went to die. I know it sounds dark, but I was in a dark place.

I just simply could not understand why this was not happening for us. During the fourth cycle, I started bargaining with God. *I will take better care of myself. I will stress less. I will have faith that He has a plan.* I started praying two to three times a day, but to no avail.

I also started realising that kids might not be part of our plan at all. It was not because we didn't want it—we wanted it more than anything else in the world. No, it was just because life sucks, as simple and as stupid as that. No real reason; the universe just doesn't feel like blessing your sorry arse with a child, but good job for being a good person; here, have a gold star. The universe, or whoever was in charge of my fate, didn't care if I was a good or bad person or how many times I prayed or went to church. No. The universe couldn't give a flying fuck about me. It just is what is, and I had to start accepting it.

Knowing this didn't change anything, and I frankly gave the universe a middle finger, deciding that I would push on and try again with another cycle. Another cycle and another egg collection because, you know, Sonja and her husband can't make embryos that want to live to day five. No, all their embryos die at day three. Maybe this was a sign that we shouldn't be parents. Maybe if you can't make a baby, it means you should not have one. Like a cruel rule created by whoever was in charge of this shitshow that was my life.

We were resetting again to the default setting of looking for answers and planning the next cycle, life just passing us by.

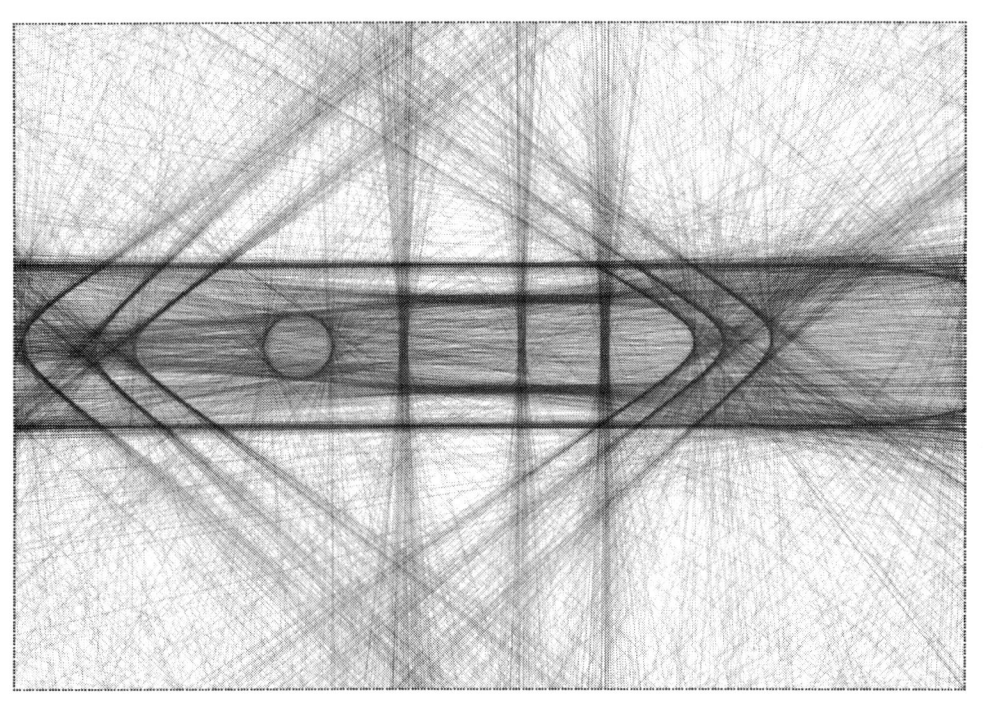

Chapter 12

WHEN IT ALL GOT TOO MUCH

IT WAS LIKE OUR lives were just running in this loop: do your cycle, fail, cry, seek solutions, try again. It was becoming extremely exhausting, physically and emotionally. How much more would we be willing to take?

Every time we failed, I would say that I couldn't do it anymore. Yet I did. Many people would wonder why you would put your body through hormone simulation and egg collection more than four times if you haven't had success. The short answer is hope. I was holding onto the only thing that had the possibility of fulfilling my dream of becoming a mother one day. I no longer cared about the injections. Sure, they still hurt a lot, but it was like I was going through life on autopilot. All I could see was the next cycle and the hope it would bring. The chance of having a family.

We took our usual break for a couple of months. I decided more than my husband that we should do a cycle in December, as late as possible. This would give the opportunity for me to be relaxed and on holiday while I was in the two-week wait. He agreed. I also wondered how many times my husband agreed because he truly believed it was the right choice and how many times he did it because he could see the hope and determination in my eyes.

After our fourth failed cycle, I realised that my mental health was deteriorating. I was erratic, extremely anxious, depressed, and angry and had outbursts and breakdowns when the most insignificant thing happened. I was out of control, and hiding it from the world was infuriating and exhausting.

I had no friends who truly understood. None of them were in this situation. They would not understand what I was feeling, would they? I did not know who to talk to and I had never found psychologists helpful, although I did try a few times during our journey.

During the course of our IVF treatment, I also spoke to a work colleague who had fertility struggles. It was nice to know that there was someone who understood. I was told that there were multiple people at my firm who actually had difficulties but obviously was not told who exactly. It would have been nice to talk to them and hear their experiences, or so I thought. It was only until later when a particular colleague talked to me about it that I realised that talking to people who successfully did IVF was not going to make me feel better. No, no, no. Instead, it made me feel worse about myself. Imagine hearing after your four failed cycles that someone did IVF just once and it worked. I would just want to tell that person to fuck off. Hearing stories of people doing IVF successfully just made me feel all the more like a failure. Why did it get to work for them and not for me? I wish there were answers.

It killed me even more when they kept telling me to hold onto hope, like I wasn't already doing that. At times, I let the thoughts creep in, only for a few minutes, that maybe I would never have kids. Thinking about it, even now, makes me a bit sad. It is like having been promised something at the start of your life; you live a good, honest life, but somehow, the promise gets broken for no reason, just because, you know, why not?

Why not take away the one thing a person has always wanted and desired? It will make them strong, some would say. Bullshit! If that is the case, then I don't want to be strong. I want to be the weakest person in the room if it means that I can have a child. Unfortunately, this was the path that was given to us, and we were trying, and failing, to suck it up.

I have this one particular bad memory and thinking about it makes me want to burst out in tears. We were doing another girls' get-together. A masseuse/nail technician person was going to come to Lily's home. I was excited, you know? I could do with a massage. I knew our pregnant friend and other friend's baby would be there, but I figured I would be okay. I could just ignore the baby and maybe sit where I couldn't see her or come close to her. This is ironic now, because I love that little girl to bits. I used this avoidance tactic over the years, although I have been getting better at being around babies on most occasions, but not all.

Anyway, I had a good cry and breakdown before the day. You know, getting it all out of my system. Just so you know, I only *thought* it was out of my system. It was still there, bubbling up slowly but surely, and it would make an appearance at the girls' day, much to my dismay.

The afternoon started fine; we were snacking and talking. Talking about whether we are doing our nails or only getting a massage done. Talking about work and what we have been up to. Normal stuff. I was fantastic to talk about normal stuff.

As mentioned, our pregnant friend was there. There was some conversation around the pregnancy. You know, the insomnia and the weird dreams, and how the insomnia actually prepares you for when you are a new mother. I wanted to yell at them to just for the love of chocolate talk about something else, but I didn't. They talked and I tried my best to zone out.

Then to my horrible surprise, someone brought baby clothes to give to the said pregnant friend. The afternoon was slowly turning into my personal hell. I was sitting there trying not to look at the baby clothes, but how could I not? It would be rude if I didn't. Yet I made no attempt to comment. Everyone was sitting there oohing and aahing over the cute baby clothes. Every time she opened up a piece of clothing, I could feel my emotions bubbling up, the tears welling up in my eyes, but I kept swallowing and blinking them away. "I will not cry; I will not cry," I kept repeating to myself.

"Oh, you are having a boy," the words came. The friend who already had a baby joked that the pregnant friend would have the difficult part at the start while she, who had a girl, was going to be facing the difficulties during the teenage years. Bubble, bubble, my emotions were getting hard to control.

How could they be so utterly insensitive? It was no secret that we were struggling, yet it was all baby talk. I am not saying hide your joy, but maybe open the presents at home.

Then the last bit of information came, that little bit that was going to push me over the edge. Setting the scene, oohing and aahing, another baby crying in the background and the words, "Sonja, I know you are doing IVF; how is that going?" Buzzer sound, wrong question, but thank you for playing. Forcing the words "not great" out of my mouth and making my way outside was my only defence. I knew it was meant as an honest and caring question, but it was all just too much. I stood outside, unable to stop the tears from falling.

Eventually Lily came out and consoled me. She asked if I wanted to go home, but I was adamant to stay there. I cried my river and went inside as if nothing had happened. It is scary to think how many times I have done this the past few years, putting on a mask just so that I would not make others uncomfortable.

That night, it occurred to me that I would need to stop the fertility treatments if the next one didn't work, but was I ready for that? The answer was a plain and simple no. Despite me not being able to recognise myself between the depression, anxiety, grief, desperation, and exhaustion, I was not ready to give up on our dream.

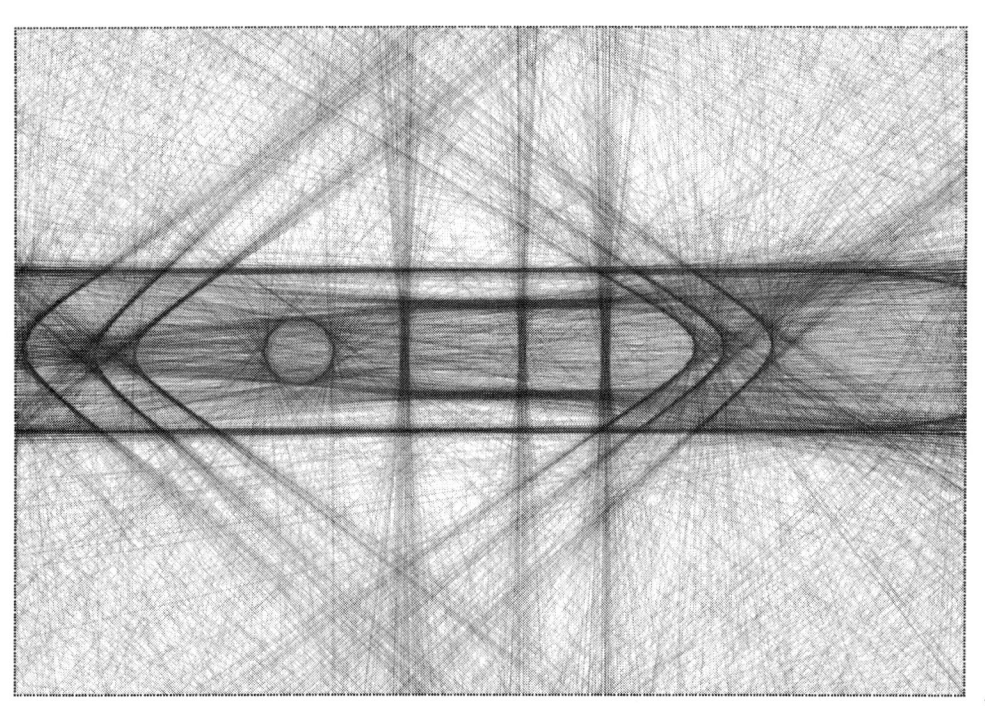

Chapter 13

THE MIRACLE

THE CYCLE IN DECEMBER started just like any other cycle. There was nothing really different except for a renewed sense of hope that I conjured up out of the ashes that were my life, an optimism I did not quite recognise. Was this the last breath I was drawing before crashing down to the reality of future childlessness? Is there some way I could use this optimism to make this cycle work? Over the course of our fertility treatments, especially this fifth one, I constantly found myself thinking, *This one will be different. This one will work. We only need one.* You know, because everyone says if you believe hard enough, it will work. I am all for believing in the power of positivity. On the other hand, I would like to see scientific evidence where merely "believing" in something made it real. Applying this concept to infertility felt silly. Believing in the Easter Bunny and Santa Claus did not make them any more real. Why, then, should it work on infertility? The answer is it shouldn't, and it probably doesn't. I believe that it is merely a coincidence that one gets pregnant by merely believing or manifesting thoughts. Maybe I am just too sceptical for this shit.

Anyway, with a renewed sense of hope and optimism, we proceeded with cycle number five, ready to walk the fine line between hope and devastation. It is quite a busy walkway, and I was a regular.

I am not going to bore you too much with all the cycle details. By this time, you know how it all goes. The biggest difference this time round was that my husband would need to go through the same surgery again to retrieve more sperm since the vials we got previously were depleted. Right after the previous cycle failed, he started seeing an adult endocrinologist, knowing that he would have to undergo the ordeal again. He did everything humanly possible to improve any chance of sperm production. Note that each time you undergo a microTESE procedure, the testicular tissue gets damaged and each time, the probability of extracting sperm is reduced, along with testicular function influenced. The treatment included high doses of HCG—yes, the pregnancy hormone, the same hormone used during IVF as the trigger—but injected daily, and he said goodbye to hot showers completely. He did this for four months straight, as the normal sperm production cycle is around three months.

The efforts were unsuccessful, with only a few much weaker sperm being found, resulting in low chance of successful fertilisation and no probability of another procedure leading to a better outcome. This was his final chance of ever having biological children of his own.

I will skip over the typical IVF cycle stuff and start when we went for the transfer. Bad news—we only got four eggs, with only one being good quality. Good news—it made it to day five. Can you believe it? It was indeed a miracle. During this transfer, I was able to see the embryo on-screen. It was an absolutely perfect blob. It was "our baby". From the moment I saw it, I got super attached it. This was it. I could feel it; this was the one that was going to stick.

It also felt like some sort of sign that we had used the last of my husband's sperm and, despite scientists telling us that the sperm was no good, it actually made a day-five embryo.

We transferred on 21 December 2021. Our blood test was due on 31 December 2021. Enter optimistic thought: *We are going to start the new year as a pregnant couple.* I was super relaxed during the two-week-wait for the first time ever, maybe it was because I knew it was going to work.

Now, I can't remember the exact day—it must have been around Christmas Eve. My husband and I were taking a walk on Coochiemudlo Island. This is a relatively small island near

Brisbane, not that that is relevant to the story. I went to the bathroom and, as I wiped, there was blood. It was different to a period. It was little spots and not a lot. Was this implantation bleeding? The hope-thermometer was rising.

Not telling my husband anything, I googled what implantation bleeding looked like. Yeah, I know, it is a bit gross, but I did not care, because it confirmed that it was implantation bleeding. Despite this, a sudden doubt had entered.

It was already four days past transfer. The embryo was supposed to implant one to two days after transfer. Late implanters result in positive pregnancies, don't they? This resulted in breaking my self-imposed two-week-wait social media ban. I had to know, was a pregnancy still in the cards, or was I out yet again? To my relief, there was a shimmer of hope—late implanter can make it.

The next day was Christmas, and all was in keep for a Christmas miracle. Everything felt extra special; it was just amazing. I was still very anxious about the late implantation and, later on, minor bleeding, so I confided in another friend. It turns out that they were also struggling to conceive and were planning on doing IVF the following year. She reassured me and wished me the best of luck. I mean, what else could she possibly do, anyway? This was out of our hands, and to my dismay, we had no control over how this was going to go.

Time ticked by slowly to the blood test day. For the first time ever, I did not take a pregnancy test. I was going to hold out until the big day. I was so sure that I was pregnant that I felt I did not need a stupid test to tell me so. Plus, tests are ridiculously expensive for something you just wee on and chuck away.

Tick, tick, tick, and then finally the day came. It was 31 December 2021. I woke up super early to get my blood tests. I nervously sat in the pathology waiting room. This was the first time I was doing the pregnancy blood test while I did not have a period. It felt good and it felt right. It was our time now. There were a few little kids waiting for their mums and I could not help but smile at their innocent faces. The idea that I was going to have one my own soon delighted me. I probably should not have been so eager.

Midday came and we were out playing a belated Christmas putt-putt with our friends. My husband once again thought that I'd would be good for us to do. We clearly did not sit on the same page of what would be good for me, but I went in anyway. What would the harm be, right? There would just be some extra people to share the joy with. Plus, the friends in question were also pregnant after a few years of struggles.

Now that I think about it, a lot—and I mean a lot—of people have gotten pregnant while we tried to conceive. It had to be about four couples, not counting acquaintances and social medial "friends". Talk about skipping the queue, people. It did not matter, though; as I said, our time had come.

Staring at the phone, I answered it, my voice a little shakier than I anticipated. I was asked whether I had time to talk. I confirmed, and then my world came crashing down like a building that was just hit by a wrecking ball. It almost felt if a wrecking ball hit me directly in the stomach. I felt nauseous and I could feel the tears welling in my eyes.

From all of this, you could probably gather that it was not the best of news; definitely not the news that I had been preparing for. I would not say it was bad news, either. It was the kind of news that puts you in limbo of how you are supposed to feel. I was pregnant, yes, but my HCG was pretty low. The pregnancy might not be viable, but there was still a chance. You know, because miracles do happen (although I do not think they were meant to happen to me; not in this lifetime, at least).

My husband could see something was wrong and I shakily gave him the news. Once again, our coping mechanisms were worlds apart. It was me who wanted to go home, be wrapped in a burrito-like blanket, and cry and my husband who wanted to continue to putt-putt and then, later that day, go to some sort of New Year's party.

How could he not see that I was not in the party mood? I suddenly was on the very fine line constantly swerving between being hopeful and breaking down. I did not really know what to feel and, most of the time, I just cried. They were not those gut-wrenching tears of sadness or disappointment that I so often cried during our IVF. These were tears of uncertainty about what was yet to come. I told a handful of people, and they sent their best wishes, everyone hoping that the "little one will stick".

The following fortnight was one of the most gruelling of my life and, to this day, I can't remember much of it. I was on autopilot, using my progesterone, you know, so I could keep this pregnancy going and googling a heap of times to try and find just that one person who also had low HCG and got their miracle. As you can imagine, I did find such people. Like I said earlier, there will also be one person.

There was hope again. Then something happened; my HCG had increased. It was still low, but it had doubled. This increased my hope again. The next few days continued in a similar fashion. I had to take a blood test every second day to see what my HCG was doing. Everything was tracking sort of normal, which was a first. I think my HCG got up to something like 102. I was still pregnant and going to be a mum.

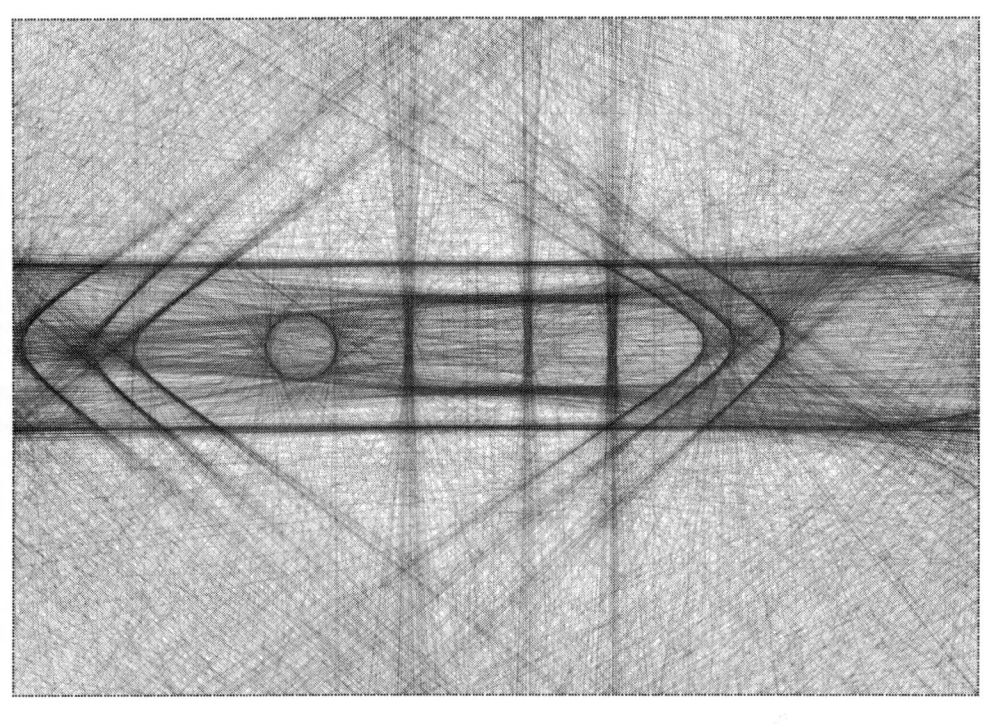

Chapter 14

PREGNANT, NOT PREGNANT

ON 10 JANUARY 2022, I was due back at work after Christmas holidays. I was feeling happy and excited, albeit nervous. I confided in a colleague. I told her that if this round did not work, we might need to throw in the towel. It was a half-hearted comment. I was still in full-on denial about what was happening.

I felt pregnant the morning of 10 January 2022, until I didn't. I started bleeding a lot. I had done some blood tests that morning after I called the clinic to ask if the bleeding was "normal". Any rational woman would have known that it was not, but I did not want to believe it. Sitting at work waiting for the call from the clinic to tell me everything was all good was nerve-racking.

My phone rang, the lady spoke, my heart started to race, and then my heart dropped into my stomach. My world turned upside down. The words, "I am sorry, dear, you have lost it," were some of the most soul-crushing words I have ever heard and, to this day, I will always remember them. I had lost our baby. Seven weeks and I lost it. Did I do something wrong? Was this my fault? Had I somehow ruined my husband's only chance to have a child with his own DNA? So many questions running through my mind, and I had zero answers. All I had to keep me company was guilt, sadness, grief, and devastation.

Right then and there I had a breakdown at work, sobbing, tears running down my face. The co-worker who I had spoken to earlier that day saw that something was wrong. All I could get out was that I had lost it. It was gone. She gave me a tight hug. I wished that her hug was enough to glue back together all the broken pieces of my heart, but it wasn't.

That day will always be embedded in my memories and heart. It will always be the one that could have been, our miracle baby that was not meant for this world. I forever wish that I had taken a pregnancy test in those early days. I was the only one to ever feel his or her presence. That way I might have had some proof that he or she existed. It was also the only opportunity that I might have had to see those iconic two pink lines, and I missed it.

Since then, I have come to hate the words "chemical pregnancy". For me, that pregnancy was as real as any other pregnancy, despite me losing it at an early stage.

Chemical pregnancy is a stupid technical word for a pregnancy that was lost very early on. They are more common than you think. If you were not actively trying to get pregnant, you might not even have realised that you were pregnant—it would be like a late period, of sorts. I, however, did know about the loss, and it was a whole different experience.

It was a one of the hardest times I have been through, but not the hardest. That was yet to come. What made this time even more difficult was the fact that my husband and I dealt with grief and loss in two very different ways. I withdrew into a bubble, and my husband just carried on like nothing had happened and it was like I had lost a dollar coin, not a baby. At least, that is what it felt like. I am pretty sure he cared and was heartbroken, too. He was just way better at compartmentalising than me.

My world had shattered. I was in disbelief, and we also had a choice to make: do we use the donor sperm or call it quits? We had gotten the worst end of the deal. We had to choose between two of the worst options. Each one of those options symbolised something we didn't want, or rather, could not imagine at that stage. It was either be childless or pursue the donor route, with the possibility that the one of us would regret the decision. Talk about being conflicted.

Now, here comes the different-people–different-approaches tizzy. Imagine a woman desperate to have a child of her own, so desperate that she is willing to use the sperm of a stranger. Then imagine a man dead set on having a child with his own DNA—which is completely understandable, yet not possible—and for him, using donor sperm is unimaginable.

We decided to take a six-month break. We needed time to think. By "we", I mainly mean my husband. I was all-in. I wanted a child, and donor sperm was the way to achieve it. Just like before, I was being selfish. I did not think about how he was feeling. I was only thinking about myself and clinging onto the only blimp of hope I had, and I was clinging on for dear life. To this day, I regret the way I handled things. I was sad, broken, hormonal, and desperate. This was not an excuse. I was not able to perceive my life without a child in it.

The next few months were filled with a lot of grief and a lot of fights. I won't bore you with all the details, as I am pretty sure you can work out for yourself what the fights were all about.

I was also stuck in this constant loop. I was see-sawing between the options, knowing what I wanted to do but not really knowing what I should do. There was also this subtle fear of losing my husband. I love him more than anything. What if we used a donor, it worked, and then it caused friction, causing us to break up? Was I really willing to gamble the possibility of losing my husband for the chance of having a child? Sadly, at that stage, the answer was yes. I truly believed that he loved me enough and would also love any child, regardless of whether it was his own blood or not. I still believe this to be true, but I am in a different space now—one where I would not gamble with our relationship.

Every few weeks, I would push my husband to talk about the donor and when we were going to do our next cycle. It was like I was an addict, addicted to hope, addicted to possibility, addicted to the idea of a family living the ideal life in their white-picket-fence homes. I wanted it all. Grief and desperation drove my thoughts and actions every minute of every day. There was nothing else in this world that mattered—not work, not friends, not hobbies. My world evolved around this child who did not even exist.

I am also sure that we lost some friends due to our infertility, or maybe it just felt that way. It was as if we were being invited to things less and less. Was it because I found it hard to be around children? Did I make people uncomfortable? Did people just not know how to deal with our situation? All of these are valid reasons, but I guess we will never truly know the why.

While dealing with this impossible choice, I was dealing with grief that no-one understood. I was grieving for something—someone that never existed and would never exist. But for me, for those few weeks, they existed. The possibility of them existed. It hurt so bad that I wanted to scream to let the pain out.

The idea that we would have children who have his eyes and my hair or my looks and his brains was torn away from us. It was torn away without any reason or explanation. There was nothing I could do or say to change it—it was just how it was. I would never have a little version of my husband and it killed me and I know it killed him even more. What killed me more was this uncanny guilt that I had. I blamed myself for losing the baby that was made with the last of his sperm. Illogical and unreasonable, yes, but it was a real feeling.

Just like that, I had started hating on my body again. *Useless body*, I would think. *What the fuck is wrong with you? Why won't you just do what you are supposed to do?* The little faith that I had in life and in God was also gone. I no longer cared if it was "all in God's plan". No, if it was His plan, it was an absolutely horrible plan, and no-one was going to tell me anything different. How could someone take away our only chance to have a 100% biological child. I don't care what Susan from church says, it was not meant to be. It did not happen for a reason, it was not God's plan, it was just shit, and everyone who had a different opinion could just fuck off.

Even worse than the above was the well-intentioned people who told me that "at least I know that I can get pregnant". I did not want to hear that; everyone was missing the point. The fact of the matter remained was that we could not have biological children. Once again, people were grasping for things to say where all they actually had to do was give me a tight hug and let me cry it out. People love to say that they are there for you if you need them, but the reality is that most people have their own life, and they can only offer you 5% even if they wanted to give you more.

So that is what happened after my early miscarriage: guilt, grief, sadness, anger, frustration, indecisiveness, conflict, depression, and anxiety, just to name a few.

I was not sure I was going to get out of this pit of unwelcome emotions, because it was starting my swallow me whole and there was no light at the end of the tunnel, just endless darkness and pain.

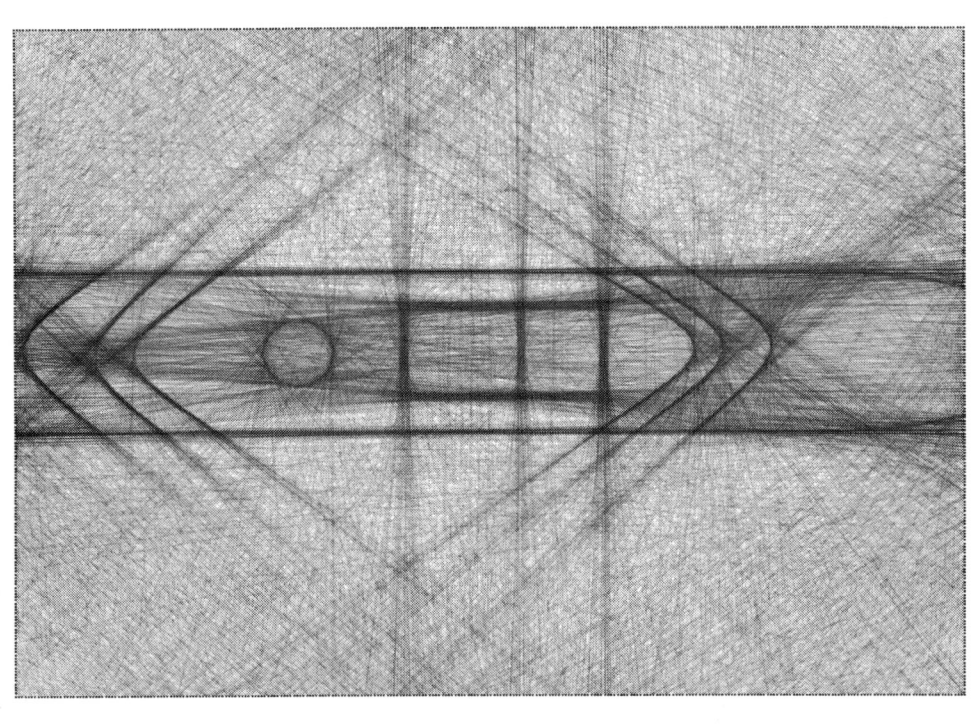

Chapter 15

THE LAST ONE

MONTHS PASSED, AUTOPILOT MODE in full swing. I remained in my dark hole, grief, pain, unfairness, and indecisiveness overwhelming me. I rarely went out. Going out with people was work. I had to put on a mask, smile, and pretend that I was not falling apart little by little. I was also losing myself a little bit day by day.

Burying myself under work, I was too busy to grieve, to think about the impossible decision that had to be made. It was work, gym, eat, sleep, repeat.

I did not seek out emotional or mental help. I was set on the belief that no-one understood or would understand. I knew zero people who had a similar journey. I was completely alone.

I could only share my feelings with my husband but, at some stage, I think even he got fed up with hearing the same feelings and arguments on repeat.

It was a broken record that went, "I want a family", "we need to use a donor", "it will still be your child", "should we do this?", "I don't know what to do", "what do you want?" On and on and on it went, until he did not want to talk about it, and then I was truly alone.

My husband felt like he was being pushed into a corner when I spoke about the donor. This was not my intention, but I can see where he got it from. My obsession, my desperation, my need for a family was growing beyond control. He wanted space to think, and I was giving him anything but. I needed an answer from him, and I needed it now.

The moment he did not want to talk about it anymore, I believed that it was over—we would not be having a child. Talk about misreading signals.

I was taking a shower one night and, all of a sudden, an overwhelming surge of emotion overcame me. Who would take care of me when I was old? What was I going to do with my life if I could not be a mother, and most importantly, who am I if I could not be a mother? I broke down. Unable to tell the difference between water and tears on my cheeks, I stood in the shower for what felt like hours.

Eventually, my husband asked what was wrong, and the record started playing again. This time, however, he did not tell me to stop, he did not shut me down. He said he had not said no to the donor, he just had not said yes yet. It was a big, life-altering decision, and he needed to think.

I was relieved to say the least but, knowing my husband and his struggles to make big decisions, I decided to put a clock on it. We were going to schedule another cycle for June 2022. He had to tell me before that if he was out.

In the months leading up to June, I tried my best not to talk to him about it, to not ask questions and to not push him, unintentionally or not. I needed him to make the right decision—that is, the decision that I wanted him to make whether it was right for him or not. On occasion, I broke the ban on talking about it with quick reminders about how children born from donors are not a bad thing and why. It was almost like a short advert promoting donors popping up at the most unsuspecting times. This was not well-received, as his expression of annoyance was pretty similar to a "fuck off". I just did not take the hint. I did not care; all I cared about was him telling me that we could go ahead and do a cycle with the donor.

Miraculously, he did. To this day, I am not 100% sure that his heart was in it. It was the most selfless thing that anybody has ever done for me, and I did not deserve it. I knew he was not 100% convinced about having donor children and his agreement to do a cycle with a donor was more because he loved me and wanted me to be happy. I say that I would have done the same thing for him, but you never know until you are in that position. That day, he gave up so much of himself, literally and figuratively, that I would never be able to thank him enough.

His selflessness gave us another chance. Look, it was not the way that I imagined my family would look, but it was still going to be a family.

There I went again hopping on the naivety horse, trotting along to destination fantasy. How could I have been so stupid after all we have been through? All he did was give us another chance, not a guarantee. I, on the other hand, was on cloud nine.

We were going to have a more unconventional family, and we could live with that. It was going to be different and hard, but it would be worth it. The very "reliable" premise I based all of our IVF cycles on was that it was all going to be worth it. "It will be worth it," she said for the sixth time. Delusional! I could almost hear my clear-minded alter ego hiding in the corner of my mind saying, *Delusional; Clearly off your rocker, you are; WTF, woman?* Just to be clear, I could almost hear her but not yet. I was ready for this cycle. I was going to own this cycle, and everything was going to work out like I envisioned it.

The latter is not exactly true. As you can gather from my story so far, IVF is not exactly something that is within your control. No, it is more like throw a dollar in a well and hoping your wish comes true because you think the goddess of fertility—who, by the way, has already screwed you over five times—has had a change of heart.

Now, getting back to the cycle, I am not going to go through the whole cycle thing again, you know this shit off by heart by now, just like me. I should just teach a class on the science of IVF and how it is bonkers. So, we do the jabs, I get violated every few days with an ultrasound, I take a nap where a bunch of guys take things out of my hoo-ha while I am sleeping, and then there we are, waiting by the phone to hear from the embryologist.

This time was different, though. It is hard to explain, but using donor sperm to fertilise my eggs made me feel like I was cheating on my husband in some weird way. I know I wasn't, but still, it was weird. Was it wrong for me to want it to work? Was it wrong for me to want another man's sperm to make me pregnant, so to speak? Saying yes out loud sounds really wrong, but that is what I wanted. Sometimes, I wondered what my husband was thinking and feeling while we waited. Did he secretly wish it not to work? I don't know, but even if he did, I would not have blamed him.

We had five mature eggs to fertilise. Yes, ladies and gentlemen, this was the best cycle if you are looking at egg count. I already took this as a sign that this cycle was going to have a good outcome. The again, I would have taken a bird pooping on my head as a good sign, too.

Have you ever played the lottery and you got each and every number right but then your heart sinks and drops into your stomach as you did not get the bonus ball? Keep that feeling in mind, but maybe exaggerate it a little bit in your mind.

The phone rings. It is either the doctor or the embryologist—I can't remember. You answer and then suddenly you fall. You fall off your horse; you get that last kick in the gut that sends you over the edge. Your heart gets broken, yet again, this time beyond repair. You did not win the lotto; you did not get the bonus ball. You got all the numbers, the right number of eggs, healthy clinically tested sperm, but the goddess of fertility has screwed you over yet again in the worst possible way.

You might wonder what type of news could have been so bad. I mean, we have had a cancelled cycle, a zero-egg cycle, OHSS, a few cycles where we only got one good egg—we even had an early miscarriage. What could possibly be so bad? I introduce to you, ladies and gentlemen, the worst news ever:

"Sorry, none of the five eggs fertilised." I did not know what to do or what to say.

It was like everything was happening in slow motion. None had fertilised. I had gone through this again for nothing. Maybe I was being punished because I forced my husband to use the donor sperm. Yes, that must be it. Why else would it not have worked?

We have now gone through this six times. Should it not have worked by now? Suddenly a harsh clarity was reaching me. Ideas clouding my judgement started to drift away slowly. I was coming to a realisation but not acceptance. Pushing all that aside, for the time being, I fell back, down, down, down, into my pit of grief that was ever-growing. I never truly allowed myself the opportunity to heal.

This time would be the last time that I might be able to claw myself out, if at all. The grief and the heartbreak was killing me from the inside. I was no longer able to recognise the person that I had become.

I can't even remember how I told my husband or what he said or did not say. Everything was just too unreal.

It is like we have been standing at the baggage claim at the airport for the past three years. The baggage of all our friends, even those on later flights, had arrived, but we were still standing at the carousel. It was going round and round, but there was no baggage to claim for us. It was never going to arrive; it was lost.

I thought that the impossible choice was the one between donor sperm and no kids, but I was wrong. The most impossible decision was whether or not to stop fertility treatments, and the time had come for us to make it.

Our doctor once again had no words and, in his sincerest manner, gave us options. We could go donor for both me and my husband, or we could pick another sperm donor and see if that worked, or if we could no longer ride this traumatic emotional roller-coaster—just stop, take a break, and see where life takes us.

I did not want to choose. Choosing had a sense of finality that I did not want. I was scared like a little child. I wanted someone to make the choice for us, but they could not. The ball was in our court. We had to choose: do we throw the ball again into the unknown and hit a home run or do we drop the ball and walk away?

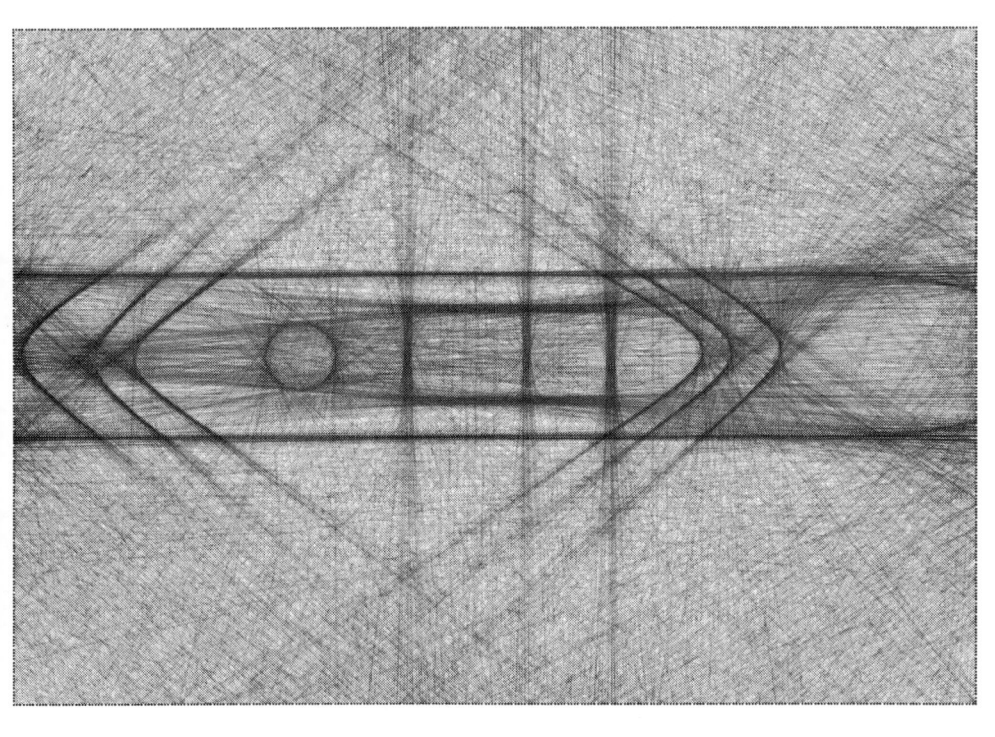

Chapter 16

OPTING OUT

YOU MIGHT WONDER HOW you make such a decision. I was in constant conflict with myself, fearing to make the wrong one. My husband was his ever-supportive self, saying that, although he did not think using a different donor would work, we could give that a go. He wanted me to decide, as he knew how hard it was for him to give up his biological link to a child.

In the next few weeks, maybe months, I did research about egg donation, how it worked, and the success rates. Spoiler alert: no success guaranteed. Thy should make that the slogan for IVF. It could say, *Struggling with infertility? Try IVF! Terms and conditions apply.*

Anyway, I was not that attached to my DNA, although it would have been great to have a little curly brown-haired girl who loved dancing, reading, and the outdoors as much as me. Someone I could go shopping, share secrets, and play dress up with. Then again, not all dreams are made to come true.

As much as I wanted to try with my eggs again, three things were holding me back. One, if IVF did not work the first six times, why would it now? Two, I knew my husband did not really want children made of donors. Three, what if it did work but I lost my husband in the process? Was it truly worth it to gamble a relationship for something that was not real? Unlike earlier, this time, I could say that it wasn't worth the gamble.

I have never told my husband how I came to make my final decision. It was about two months after my knee surgery, and I was talking to a friend who asked how IVF was going. I do my best reasoning when I talk to people about my thoughts and feelings and how I got there. As I was talking to a friend at a barbecue, I realised that, deep down, I had already made the choice, but I was afraid to say it out loud.

I no longer wanted to ride the emotional roller-coaster. I no longer wanted to fight with my husband about whether we should use donors or when our next IVF cycle should be. I no longer wanted to live in a world where I was so grief-stricken that I changed as a person. I no longer wanted to spend thousands of dollars and get nothing back but heartbreak. I no longer wanted to live in a world where I expected my husband to make a selfless choice because I was being selfish about what I wanted. I just wanted everything to stop and be okay. Unfortunately, making the choice to no longer pursue fertility treatments is easier said than done. I have come to the realisation, but now I had to speak up.

That night we got home around maybe 11 pm. My heart was weighing heavy, but I knew it was time. I stood in the bathroom, already having washed all my make up off my face. I called my husband.

I remember feeling super nervous and sad about what I was about to say. It was gonna hurt. Just typing this is making me cry.

I said to him that I wanted to tell him something, but I needed him to let me talk without interruption, as I needed to get something off my heart and chest. I knew that if he interrupted me, I would lose my courage and swallow my words, swallow the reality which both of us were too afraid to say out loud or even think.

"I don't think we should try again." My throat felt tight as I said those words. After that, everything tumbled out of my mouth. I told him that if IVF was meant to work for us, it would have. I said that I knew that he was not 100% sold on the donor idea and I was tired of pushing him and honestly tired of grieving and feeling like I was drowning. I was scared that if the IVF worked with a donor, he would resent me and the child and I would lose him, and I would not be able to live with that, as I just loved him too much. I said I knew that the next cycle might work, but it also might not. I said that I wanted to move forward knowing all that we do and all that we don't and forge a new life for us. I wanted us to go back to our former selves, or at least a version of them. The ones who were happy for the most part. We have been tainted by grief, unfairness, trauma, and heartbreak, and that has changed us. We will never be 100% who we were, but we could be happy again. It might not happen overnight, and it will take probably a lot of years, but I believed that we could be happy without children.

The words just flowed. I told him I knew in my heart that he would have been an amazing dad. He would always have been present and helped this little person grow into an amazing human being. I also know that I would have been a great mother.

Unfortunately, life is not fair and not all dreams are made to come true. It does not matter how much you hope or pray or how many positive vibes someone sends you. It does not matter how loud you scream out to the universe that you are ready to be parents. Sometimes, it just is was it is. I don't think our inability to have children happened for a reason, and I don't think that it was God's plan. It just happened and we needed to find a way to navigate it individually but also as a couple.

I could see the pain and the sadness in his eyes, but he knew where I was coming from, and he, too, knew it was time to move on.

What happens happens, and then we die. There does not have to be a reason for everything. Some things just are.

I think I talked out my heart that night for something close to ten to fifteen minutes, or at least it felt that way. I could have kept going for hours—in the end, it all would have boiled down to the same thing. It was the end, and we were opting out of fertility treatments.

That night was followed by multiple breakdowns and me questioning whether we were making the right choice.

I distinctly remember one weekend: I sat in the spare bedroom on the floor. I had lost my shit again. I had packed up all the teddy bears and children's books that I collected over the years and also those my mum left me when she died. I could no longer look at them. The spare room was meant to be our child's room. Every inch of that room was filled with reminders of something that I was never going to have.

I was never going to be able to experience how it felt to reveal to my husband that I was carrying a little version of us inside me. I was never going to experience how it felt to carry life inside me. I was never going to experience how it felt like to bring life into this world or to have a little human being dependent just on us to keep him or her alive. I was never going to be able to see a little version of me grow up and help him or her along the way. I was never going to be able to go to sports games or wipe away tears or share excitement. There will be no first step pictures. There will be no first day of school or first day of college pictures. All I could see was an endless row of empty photo frames where our children were supposed to be.

There is an endless list of things that we are missing out on just because life sucks. That day, in the same spare room that is now my office, I packed all our children's books and goodies in a bag. I felt like having them and seeing them was a reminder of what I will never have but it also, at least for me, symbolised hope. Hope that, maybe, one day, by some miracle, we would get pregnant, and I was so tired of hoping that I just could not do it anymore.

It broke my heart into pieces when we gave away all of those things to a friend who had recently had a baby. I kept the one book I mentioned in the beginning—the one where my mum had written *To my grandchild, love Grandma R.* I could not throw it away. I also have two teddy bears my mum had made for me while she was alive. They are the most beautiful white teddies. I am keeping them in the closet and one day I would like to take them out and put them in a room somewhere. For me they are Daxton and Peyton, the children I carry in my heart but who were not destined for this world. I am not ready for that yet so, for now, they are neatly packed away in plastic so they are protected until the day comes when I am ready. I might never be.

My husband found me on the floor of the spare room that day. He tried to talk me into keeping everything and maybe placing it in storage, but I couldn't. I knew the dream was dead.

We sat in that room for maybe an hour, maybe more. We cried, we talked about it, we cried some more, we held each other, and we cried until there were no more tears left. Well, the tears had dried up for the day and we were just exhausted.

We had finally made the choice. The choice to no longer hope, wait, and then be slammed into a wall at hyper speed. I also made the choice because I did not want to go my entire life waiting and hoping for something to happen while life and all the beautiful things it had to offer passed me buy. More importantly, I made the choice because I love my husband more than anything in this world and I cannot imagine a life without him because I was being irrational, desperate, and selfish.

We were afraid, and who could blame us? We were about to embark on a life that we did not plan. In no version of reality is this what we wanted, but it is what we got. I did not know where to start. I did not know who I was if not a mum. The only consolation was that I was not alone in it.

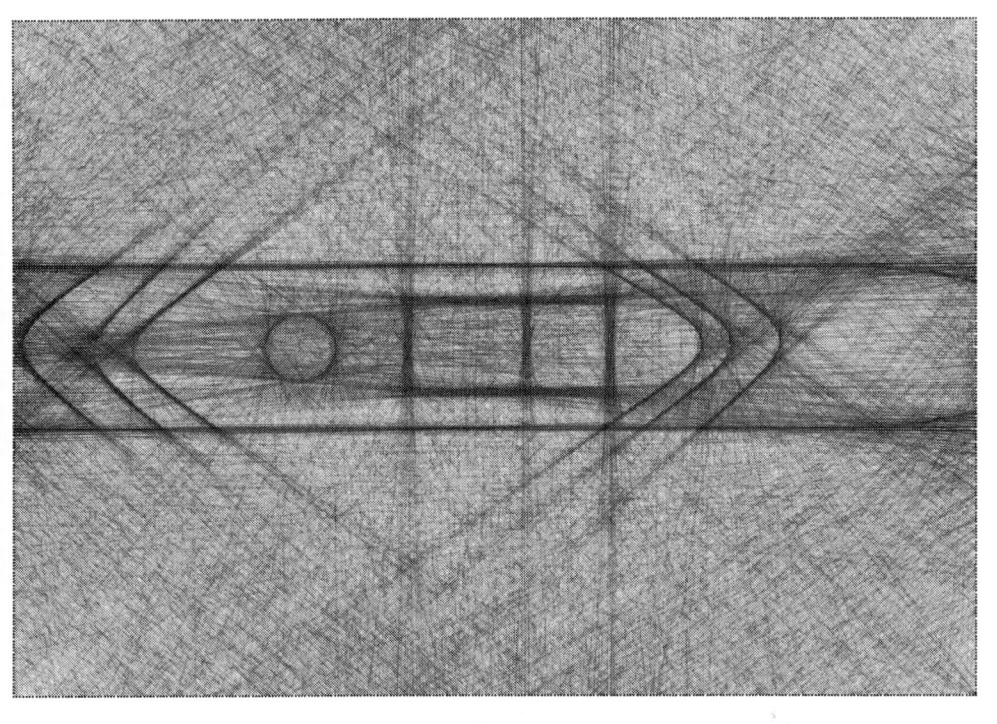

Chapter 17

CHILDLESS NOT BY CHOICE

IT HAS BEEN ABOUT a year since we pulled the plug. Sometimes, I stop in my tracks to watch a small child running to their mother and giving them a big hug. The sight overwhelms me with sadness.

I have lost friends during our journey. It might be all my fault, it might not. I was not equipped to deal with them having children or having babies or having baby talk around me. They would all say that they can't imagine how hard it must be to go through infertility and consequent childlessness, yet baby talk is not toned down. I do not expect people to manage my triggers; my triggers are my responsibility. I do, however, expect people to exhibit sensitivity and compassion. I expect people to not make a situation harder for others than it already is.

I engage with babies on my own terms now. I will walk away when I am uncomfortable. I will say "No, I do not want to hold your baby. Why? Because it will make me cry." The feebly glued pieces of my heart break a lot of the time when I see a simple pregnancy announcement. I am pretty sure it will always be hard; I will just get better at dealing with it.

My heart still breaks when someone at works sends a sonogram around or announces a pregnancy. I feel like an outsider when people talk about their children at work and in my personal life. I have nothing to contribute to the conversation and I definitely do not run to go and see the new baby that is visiting the office. I run in the opposite direction.

Mother's Day is my least favourite day of the year. My mother has passed on, and we can't have children. It is just a reminder of all that I have lost and all that I will never be or have. Some would say that I should not see it in such negative light, but I have no other way to see it in this moment in time.

I constantly tell people I am fine about making the decision, and most of the time, I am. However, there are still a lot of times when my grief sneaks up on me.

It is safe to say that, so far, it has not been easy. I have good moments and hard moments.

We are childless not by choice, and there are a lot of us out there. Those of us who are childless due to failed IVF, like us, and those who are childless due to circumstance or illness or whatever the case may be. All of us have our own stories, and all of us matter, even though we are not parents. There is more to life than being a mother, but because society has indoctrinated us into the whole marriage-and-kids thing, it is hard to imagine a life where a person does not have it and many people would tell you it is "weird". An elderly lady once told me that not having children takes away the value that your life brings. I could not disagree more. Initially, I thought that I was supposed to live some sort of extravagant life just because I could not have kids, but I don't—I just need to be happy.

For now, I am counting my blessings. I am blessed with an amazing husband who stood next to me through everything. I have a great workplace. I have friends who know about our childlessness not by choice, and they do not ask questions or talk about it unless we bring it up. They don't make life more difficult than it has to be.

I made a conscious decision to do things I love, like writing stories, going for walks, hiking, reading more, and travelling. I am also trying to focus on all the things I can do without kids. I can travel. I can sleep in late on weekends. I can have naked Sundays if I want to. I can eat chocolate and popcorn for dinner and so much more. Sure, many would say it is second prize, but so what? This is what keeps me going. I am as happy as one can be in such a situation, and I am healing.

It has not been easy, and truth be told, I will always have a little Peyton-and-Daxton-shaped hole in my heart. I will carry my disenfranchised grief with me until the end of time, but I will grow with it, and one day, I will wake up and it will still be there, but it will be less debilitating.

Did we make the wrong choice? I guess we will never know. Our life has made a 360-degree spin. I can no longer see myself pursuing IVF, surrogacy, adoption, or foster care. Everyone always says how having children changes your life, but no-one ever talks about how your life changes when you can't have kids.

Trying to start a family has taken a good three years of my life away, but despite this, I would not change a thing. Failed IVF is part of our story now, and we would not be who we are today if it was not for it. I am more resilient. It gave me perspective of the reality of life and, most importantly, it has given me a stronger marriage.

We are now embarking on a new journey—a journey that is a whole lot different than we had planned ten years ago. It is uncharted territory, it is scary, and I do not know what the hell I am doing half of the time. It is now my time to find out who I am if not a mother. It is a journey to find what makes me happy. It will probably be a rocky road at times, but I am going to make the best of it. I have only one life, and I need to live it, and I am lucky enough to be able to do it with one of the most remarkable, selfless men at my side.

Acknowledgements

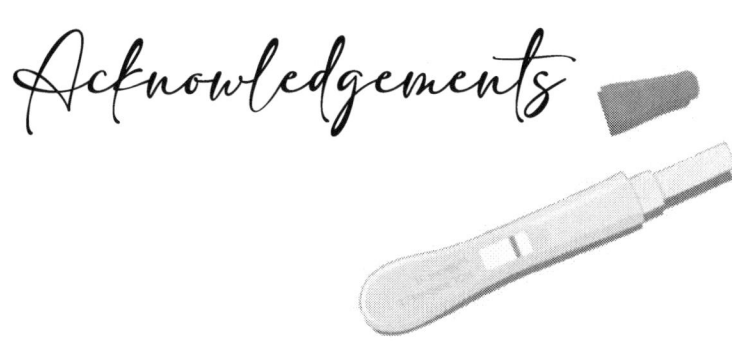

I WANT TO THANK my husband for walking this rocky, pothole-filled, earthquake-ridden path with me and also for him still being there after all that has happened. I also want to thank him for encouraging me to write this book.

I want to thank my friends and colleagues. You know who you are—you listened to the same stories and rants over and over again and provided a shoulder to cry on my when husband's shoulder was too heavy.

I want to thank my family for being so supportive, even when you didn't know what to say or didn't say anything at all.

I also want to thank our doctor, who tried everything in his medical power to help us bring a life into this world, and the nurses and other medical staff for your compassion and empathy.

My workplace deserves a shout-out, as they have been so supporting through this process.

I am not sure I would have survived this journey if it was not for all of you, so thank you from the bottom of my heart for your love and never-ending support. I love you all, and I am grateful that I can share this new chapter with you.

Printed in Great Britain
by Amazon